YOU GOT SOME NERVE

Eye of Heru

Chase Duquesnay EnQi ReaL

Amazon

Copyright © 2024 Chase Duquesnay

All rights reserved

The characters and events portrayed in this book are fictitious. Any similarity to real persons, living or dead, is coincidental and not intended by the author. None of the books in these series are written with the intent to be Medical in any shape form or fashion. These books are strictly for edutainment.

No part of this book may be reproduced, or stored in a retrieval system, or transmitted in any form or by any means, electronic, mechanical, photocopying, recording, or otherwise, without express written permission of the publisher.

ISBN: 9798322042815

Cover design by: EnQi ReaL

Printed in the United States of America

This one is for us, those who are against the antelope people.

CONTENTS

INTRODUCTION

This introduction may not be to a beginning, but a ending... We may need to start a new series...

The Electrician Series...

IGNORANT REGGIE

God (the Sun) speaks (emits radio waves) that you hear (absorb and convert) through your antenna (**the spine**). The nerves help distribute this information to the Plasma based Crystal disc, fitted with integrated circuits as well as gates and channels.

How can the eye of Heru and the Djed Pillar be so well known and yet I get attacked for discovering that the Was Scepter is the Aorta?

The following article from the National Library of Medicine further incinerates the claims made by Dr. Clark & Leonard Jeffries student Reginald A. Mabry. How were the Ancient Egyptians able to name the spine, vertebrae, meninges & spinal fluid without studying the Anatomy? It's about time we say to Reggie and the Race Hustlers like him...

You got some Nerve!!!

Chapter 3: neurology in ancient Egypt

George K York 3rd 1, David A Steinberg
Affiliations expand

- PMID: 19892106 DOI: 10.1016/S0072-9752(08)02103-9

Abstract

Neurology, in the modern sense, did not exist in ancient Egypt, where medicine was a compound of natural, magical and religious elements, with different practitioners for each form of healing. Nevertheless, Egyptian doctors made careful observations of illness and injury, some of which involved the nervous system. Modern scholars have three sources of information about Egyptian medicine: papyri, inscriptions, and mummified remains. **These tell us that the Egyptians had words for the skull, brain, vertebrae, spinal fluid and meninges, though they do not say if they assigned any function to them**. They described unconsciousness, quadriparesis, hemiparesis and dementia. We can recognize neurological injuries, such as traumatic hemiparesis and cervical dislocation with paraplegia, in the well known Edwin Smith surgical papyrus. Similarly recognizable in the Ebers papyrus is a description of migraine. An inscription from the tomb of the vizier Weshptah, dated c. 2455 BCE, seems to describe stroke, and Herodotus describes epilepsy in Hellenistic Egypt. We have very little understanding of how Egyptian physicians organized these observations, but we may learn something of Egyptian culture by examining them. At the same time, modern physicians feel some connection to Egyptian physicians and can plausibly claim to be filling a similar societal role.

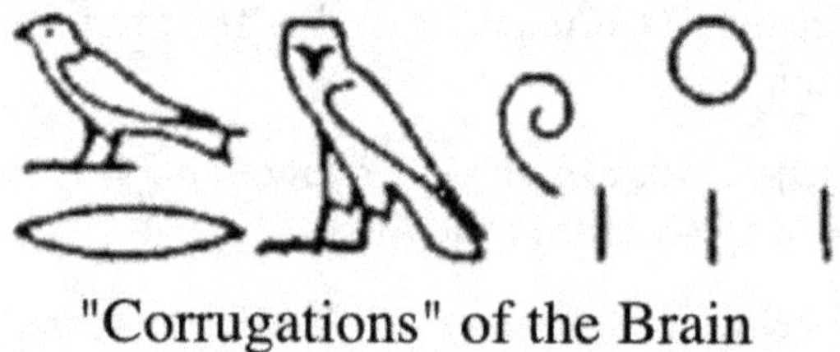

"Corrugations" of the Brain

Corrugations - Wrinkles, Waves or Grooves "like those corrugations

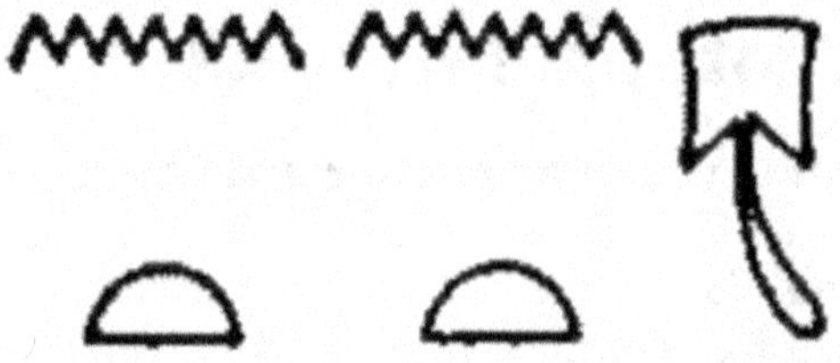

"Membrane" enveloping the Brain

which form molten copper".

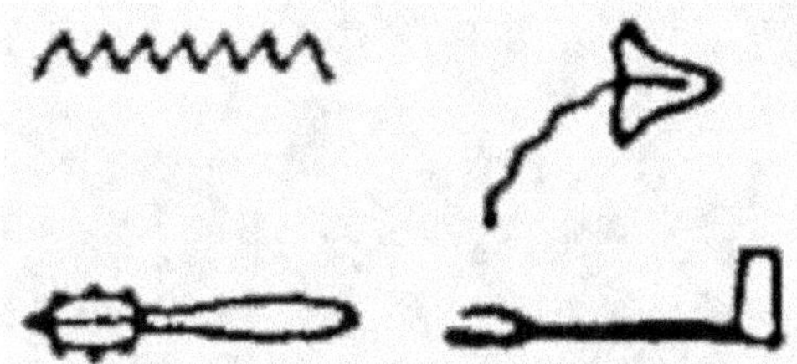

"Fluid" in the Interior of the Head

"Coverings of the Brain."

Cerebral Spinal Fluid

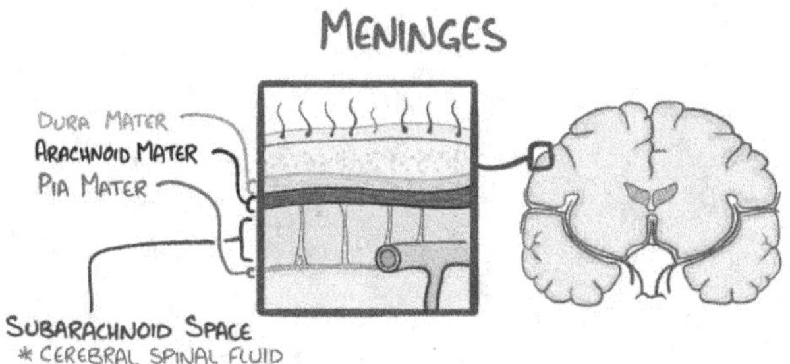

Goat Time...

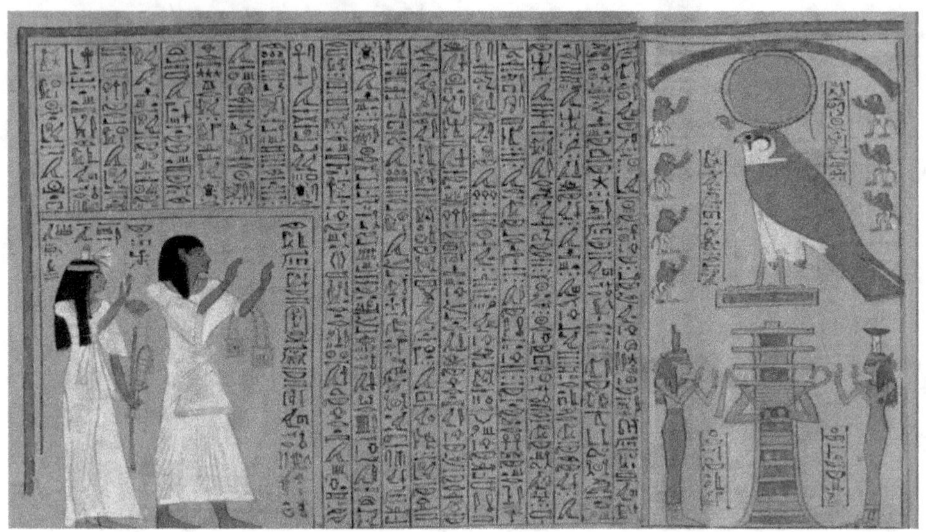

Figures adoring Ra-Horakhty, New Kingdom (ca. 1292-1189 BCE), via the British Museum

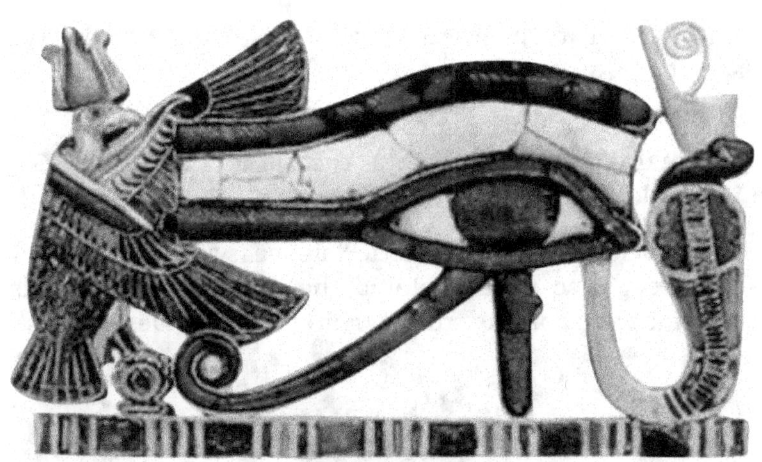

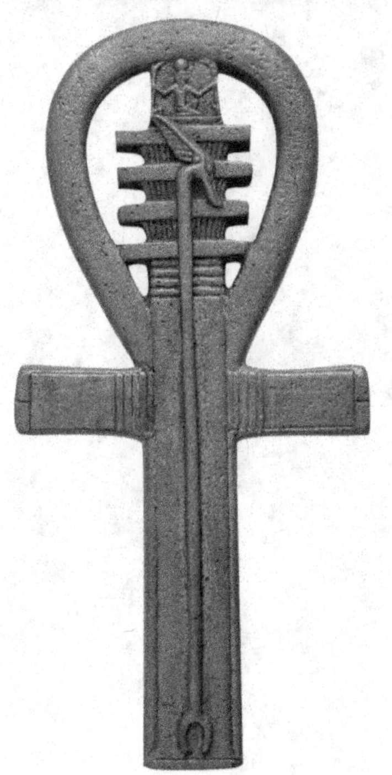

We have the Dr. EnQi Totem, its the Ankh, Was, Djed, Nekhbet & Shen, Eye of Heru & the Naga.

We have decoded these as the Reproductive System symbolic of Electromagnetism (male/female), the Aorta, the Spine, Rebirth & HGT, the Brain & 3rd Ventricle.

The prevailing ideology surrounding Kemetic Science is that the Ancient Egyptians were too stupid to have explored the human body. This is would be shameful if it were coming from "Whitefolks" or "Desertfolks",

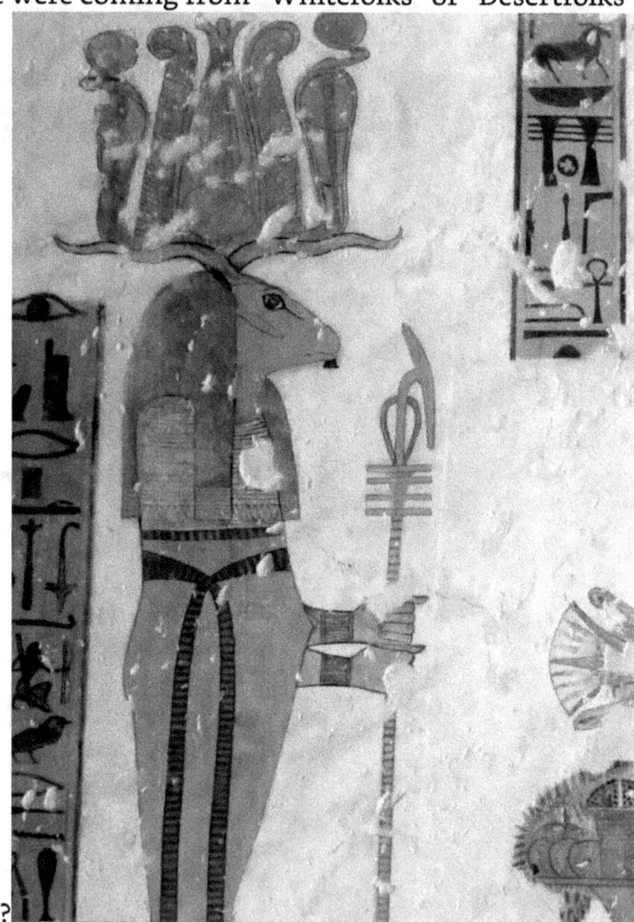

but from "Blackfolks"?!?

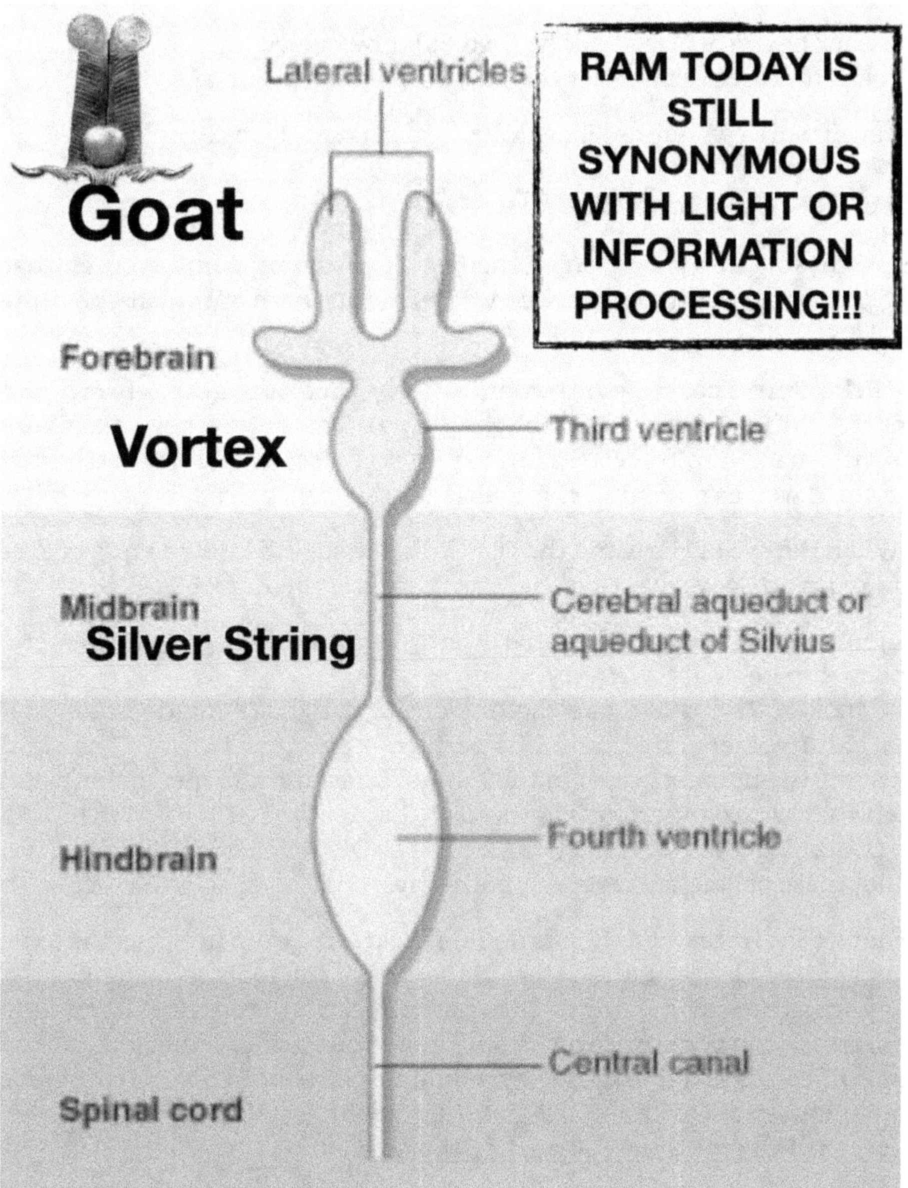

You got some Nerve!!!

God (the Sun) speaks (emits radio waves) that you hear (absorb and convert) through your antenna (**the spine**). The nerves help distribute this information to the Plasma based Crystal disc, fitted with integrated circuits as well as gates and channels.

How can the eye of Heru and the Djed Pillar be so well known and yet I get attacked for discovering that the Was Scepter is the Aorta?

It is even worse when the "Blackfolks" are trusted "Black Scholars"!!!

You got some Nerve!!!

These guys make a living off of the Legacy of the men and women that gave the world Math and Science while calling them stupid at the same time!!!

God (the Sun) speaks (emits radio waves) that you hear (absorb and convert) through your antenna (**the spine**). The nerves help distribute this information to the Plasma based Crystal disc, fitted with integrated circuits as well as gates and channels.

How can the eye of Heru and the Djed Pillar be so well known and yet I get attacked for discovering that the Was Scepter is the Aorta?

Dr. John Henrik Clarke & Leonard Jeffries via their Legacy in Kemetic Scholarship Reginald A. Mabry
have spoken. They have said the Ancient Egyptians (Kemetic Scientists) only had tweezers and could not perform anatomical study. The skull has some the hardest bones in the human body, if these men believe and teach that is was not possible to view the Aorta, THEN IT WOULD BE IMPOSSIBLE TO VIEW THE PINEAL GLAND OR THE 3RD VENTRICLE! Do not let these people try to have it both ways.

Do not let the Antelope Scholars double back! If they did not have the tools to recognize the Aorta, then they did not have the tools to recognize the inner structures of the brain. The mummification process will not help them either, the brain was supposedly pulled out through the nose during mummification. That means they would not have been able to recognize the structures of the brain after, pulling the brain out through it's nose. <u>This is the Fall of the Black Kemetic Scholars</u>.

THE NERVE OF SOME PEOPLE

The human body is estimated to have over 7 trillion nerves on average! Over 40,000 of these nerves are located in or directly attached to the Heart.

On average we have over 45 miles of the most efficient electrical wiring known to man.

In the Race Hustler series, particularly book #5, which is also book #1 of the True & Living Kemetic Science series, we discuss the electronic nature of the body. Please read or reread that book.

The Heart almost as packed with Neurons as it is with Melanocytes. In fact the skin has the most Melanocytes and accordingly has the most nerves! Melanocytes and Nerves/Neurons come from the same germ layers.

God (the Sun) speaks (emits radio waves) that you hear (absorb and convert) through your antenna (**the spine**). The nerves help distribute this information to the Plasma based Crystal disc, fitted with integrated circuits as well as gates and channels.

How can the eye of Heru and the Djed Pillar be so well known and yet I get attacked for discovering that the Was Scepter is the Aorta?

You got some Nerve!!!

God (the Sun) speaks (emits radio waves) that you hear (absorb and convert) through your antenna (**the spine**). The nerves help distribute this information to the Plasma based Crystal disc, fitted with integrated circuits as well as gates and channels.

How can the eye of Heru and the Djed Pillar be so well known and yet I get attacked for discovering that the Was Scepter is the Aorta?

You got some Nerve!!!

The trillions of Computer Chips you have in your Electronic Body are wired by these nerves. How is it possible that the spine is known by Kemetic Scientist and not it's make up? The spine is the **Motherboard**, I almost labeled it a <u>backplane</u>. The difference is the connection to the waveguide we detail in the Movement book so we won't bore you with those details here... The spine not only is the hub for all the electrical wiring it produces blood!

What is a nerve cell or neuron?

The first thing we need to know is that these cells are the exact opposite of their twin. Melanocytes and Neurons are Fraternal Twins. The Melanocytes is designed to absorbs electromagnetic waves and Neurons are designed to create electromagnetic waves.

- **Cell body:** Similar to the other Computer Chips in your System, organelles the nucleus etc...

- **Dendrites:** Dendrites are specific antenna that only pick up the incoming signals of other neurons.

- **Axon:** This is another specialized antenna and is usually larger than a dendrite. This antenna is insulated by a specialized material called myelin to protect the signal and chemical conversion of light. This is the antenna that produces out going signals.

How?

1. Neurons create an electromagnetic impulse which is sent down the length of the axon. By the end of the axon the electromagnetic signal is converted into a chemicals. These groups of Khemicals are grouped together as molecules, the molecules are called neurotransmitters.

2. Neurotransmitters are released into space between the axon and dendrite called a synapse.

3.   When Neurotransmitters bind to dendrites the chemical signal is converted back into an electricomagnetic signal and travels the length of the neuron.

The major difference between Nerves and Neurons is that nerves are just thought about by their body. Axons of are bundled together to make them thicker. Axons being bundled together helps the CNS (axons are called tracts) and PNS (peripheral nerves) communicate.

The skin, rich in Melanocytes is complemented by Nerves however the Bone home of the Stem Cells is almost as highly wired!

In practical medicine only two groups of nerves are primary focus, Cranial Nerves and Spinal Nerves. The cranial nerves are located on the bottom of the brain. We have 12 pair of cranial nerves and 31 pair of spinal nerves, interestingly enough the 62 nerves is close to the 61 codons (plus 3 stop codons).

Wiki explain the cranial nerves very simply:
- The terminal nerve (0), is a thin network of fibers associated with the dura and lamina terminalis running rostral to the olfactory nerve, with projections through the cribriform plate.
- The olfactory nerve (I), passes through perforations in the cribriform plate part of the ethmoid bone. The nerve fibres end in the upper nasal cavity.
- The optic nerve (II) passes through the optic foramen in the sphenoid bone as it travels to the eye.
- The oculomotor nerve (III), trochlear nerve (IV), abducens nerve (VI) and the ophthalmic branch of the trigeminal nerve (V1) travel through the cavernous sinus into the superior orbital fissure, passing out of the skull into the orbit.
- The maxillary division of the trigeminal nerve (V2) passes through foramen rotundum in the sphenoid bone.
- The mandibular division of the trigeminal nerve (V3) passes through foramen ovale of the sphenoid bone.
- The facial nerve (VII) and vestibulocochlear nerve (VIII) both enter the internal auditory canal in the temporal bone. The facial nerve then reaches the side of the face by using the stylomastoid foramen, also in the temporal bone. Its fibers then spread out to reach and control all of the muscles of facial expression. The vestibulocochlear nerve reaches the organs that control balance and hearing in the temporal bone and therefore does not reach the

external surface of the skull.

-     The glossopharyngeal (IX), vagus (X) and accessory nerve (XI) all leave the skull via the jugular foramen to enter the neck. The glossopharyngeal nerve provides sensation to the upper throat and the back of the tongue, the vagus supplies the muscles in the larynx and continues downward to supply parasympathetic supply to the chest and abdomen. The accessory nerve controls the trapezius and sternocleidomastoid muscles in the neck and shoulder.

    ·

-     Schematic 3D model of the cranial nerves
-     The hypoglossal nerve (XII) exits the skull using the hypoglossal canal in the occipital bone.

The Spinal Cord is grouped into 5 for simplicity:

-     C1-C8: These are cervical or neck nerves, they control neck movement, feeling in your hands, and diaphragm movement for breathing.
-     T1-T12: The thoracic nerves are in the chest. They are primarily for the chest and ab muscle, they also contribute to the feeling of the skin on the chest and back.
-     L1-L5: These lumbar nerves or lower back nerves control the movement and feeling in the hips and legs.
-     S1-S5: Sacral nerves in the pelvis govern the bowels, bladder control, and sexual function.
-     Coccygeal nerves: Base of the spine, carry feeling from the skin around the tailbone area.

Nerve impulses have a net change of about 110 millivolts on average across the axon's membrane. These impulses travel at 100 metros per second. These electromagnetic waves of nerves and neurons produce over 100 different molecules, this is the language of Neurons and Nerves.

The basal or basic electrical rhythm (BER) or electrical control activity (ECA) is the spontaneous depolarization and repolarization of pacemaker cells known as interstitial cells of Cajal (ICCs) in the smooth muscle of the stomach, small intestine, and large intestine. This electrical rhythm is spread through gap junctions in the smooth muscle of the GI tract.[1] These pacemaker cells, also called the ICCs, control the frequency of contractions in the gastrointestinal tract. The cells can be located in either the circular or longitudinal layer of the smooth muscle in the GI tract; circular for the small and large intestine, longitudinal for the stomach.[2] The frequency of contraction differs at each location in the GI tract beginning with 3 per minute in the stomach, then 12 per minute in the duodenum, 9 per minute in the ileum, and a normally low one contraction per 30 minutes in the large intestines that increases 3 to 4 times a day due to a phenomenon called mass movement. [2] The basal electrical rhythm controls the frequency of contraction but additional neuronal and hormonal controls regulate the strength of each contraction.

Smooth muscle within the GI tract causes the involuntary peristaltic motion that moves consumed food down the esophagus and towards the rectum.[1] The smooth muscle throughout most of the GI tract is divided into two layers: an outer longitudinal layer and an inner circular layer.[1] Both layers of muscle are located within the muscularis externa. The stomach has a third layer: an innermost oblique layer.

The physical contractions of the smooth muscle cells can be caused by action potentials in efferent motor neurons of the enteric nervous system, or by receptor mediated calcium influx.[1] These efferent motor neurons of the enteric nervous system are cholinergic and adrenergic neurons.[2] The inner circular layer is innervated by both excitatory and inhibitory motor neurons, while the outer longitudinal layer is innervated by mainly excitatory neurons. These action potentials cause the smooth muscle cells to contract or relax, depending on the particular stimulation the cells receive. Longitudinal muscle fibers depend on calcium influx into the cell for excitation-contraction coupling, while circular muscle fibers rely on intracellular calcium release. Contraction of the smooth muscle can occur when the BER reaches its plateau (an absolute value less than -45mV)[citation needed] while a simultaneous stimulatory action potential occurs. A contraction will not occur unless an action potential occurs. Generally, BER waves stimulate action potentials and action potentials stimulate contractions.

- wiki

You got some Nerve!!!

God (the Sun) speaks (emits radio waves) that you hear (absorb and convert) through your antenna (**the spine**). The nerves help distribute this information to the Plasma based Crystal disc, fitted with integrated circuits as well as gates and channels.

How can the eye of Heru and the Djed Pillar be so well known and yet I get attacked for discovering that the Was Scepter is the Aorta?

FAT

Lets start a new way of thinking about exercises, exercise is not just for building muscle or losing fat, its primarily for nerve firing. Nerves actually control muscles and fat cells (all cells).

This maybe slightly out of place but nerves are also the Pain network. Pain is the healing signal, it overrides other signals. Pain tells your brain and heart exactly what is need to repair the damaged or inflamed cells. The only reason I am saying this here is because the is the reason why exercise helps moderate and in some cases obliterate pain. Back to fat, autophagy and diabetes...

MCH neurons depolarize in response to high glucose concentrations. [5] This mechanism seems to be related to glucose being used as a reactant to form ATP, which also causes MCH neurons to depolarize. [5] The neurotransmitter, glutamate, also causes MCH neurons to depolarize, while another neurotransmitter, GABA, causes MCH neurons to hyperpolarize.[5] Orexin also depolarizes MCH neurons.[5] MCH neurons seems to have an inhibitory response to MCH, but does not cause the neurons to become hyperpolarized.[5] Norepinephrine has an inhibitory effect on MCH neurons as does acetylcholine.[5] MCH neurons hyperpolarize in response to serotonin.[5] Cannabinoids have an excitatory effect on MCH neurons.[5]
Some research has shown that dopamine has an inhibitory effect on MCH neurons, but further research is needed to fully characterize this interaction.

MCH and the hormone orexin have an antagonistic relationship with one another with regards to the sleep cycle, with orexin being almost entirely active during wake periods and MCH being more active during sleep periods.[3][1] MCH also promotes sleep, and within a sleep period increased levels of MCH seem to increase the amount of time spent in REM sleep and slow waves sleep.[3] Increased levels of MCH can also increase the amount of time spent in both REM and NREM, which in turn increases total sleep duration.[3] Increased levels of sugar promotes MCH and its effect on sleep and conserving energy.

An increased presence of MCH can cause increased eating levels and has been linked to an increase in body mass.[6] Inversely, a decrease in the amount of MCH present can cause decreased levels in eating.[6] Increased amounts of MCH in olfactory regions, among others, have also been linked to an increased intake of fatty foods with high caloric content.[6] [1] Food that is found to taste good also seems to promote MCH, which reinforces the eating of that food.[1] Sugar, specifically glucose, seems to promote MCH's role in sleep and energy conservation.[1] This promoting of energy conservation has also been linked to higher body mass even when diet is controlled. - wiki

Let's roll the cheat codes out first...

Heme (RBC/Mitochondrial) Efficiency - Leptin Function

Poor Heme (RBC/Mitochondrial) Efficiency -
Electron Leakage/Inflammation

Vit A - Regulates UCP1 (Thermogenin) Function/Leptin Function

Bluelight Toxicity - Depletes Vit A/Destroying Leptin Sensitivity

Poor **Leptin** Function Boost WAT and Estrogen

Melanin Concentrating Hormone controls
Leptin, they inhibit one another!

*5 Major Mineral Elements & 60+ Micro Mineral Elements

<u>4 Fat Soluble Vitamins - Fat is not the same devoid of these Vitamins!!!</u>

Vitamin A is particularly crucial in Fat Management!

9 Water Soluble Vitamins

All Amino Acids

EFAs - EPA, DHA, ALA, LA, GLA, OA, PA & VA

Plant Pigments All Colors

Natural Lighting

Exercise - Mitochondrial Density Raises Oxygen/

VO2 Max which burns Fat

"Fat" People Are Starving!!! Nutrient Deficiency
+ Parasites Drives Cravings

The Role of Melanin-Concentrating Hormone and Its Receptors in Energy Homeostasis

Douglas J. MacNeil[1],*
Author information Article notes Copyright and License information PMC Disclaimer

Go to:

Abstract

Extensive studies in rodents with melanin-concentrating hormone (MCH) have demonstrated that the neuropeptide hormone is a potent orexigen. Acutely, MCH causes an increase in food intake, while chronically it leads to increased weight gain, primarily as an increase in fat mass. Multiple knockout mice models have confirmed the importance of MCH in modulating energy homeostasis. Animals lacking MCH, MCH-containing neurons, or the MCH receptor all are resistant to diet-induced obesity. These genetic and pharmacologic studies have prompted a large effort to identify potent and selective MCH receptor antagonists, initially as tool compounds to probe pharmacology in models of obesity, with an ultimate goal to identify novel anti-obesity drugs. In animal models, MCH antagonists have consistently shown efficacy in reducing food intake acutely and inhibiting body-weight gain when given chronically. Five compounds have proceeded into clinical testing. Although they were reported as well-tolerated, none has advanced to long-term efficacy and safety studies.

Keywords: MCH, neuropeptide, MCHR1, orexigenic, obesity, KO mice, antagonist, clinical study

Go to:

Introduction

The mammalian form of melanin-concentrating hormone (MCH), is a 19-amino acid cyclic peptide encoded within a 165-amino acid preprohormone (Figure

(Figure1)

1) (Vaughan et al., 1989). MCH has been associated with a wide variety of behaviors (see recent reviews by Saito and Nagasaki, 2008; Antal-Zimanyi and Khawaja, 2009; Chung et al., 2011), but the focus of this review is the role of MCH in energy homeostasis. The amino acid sequence of MCH is identical in all mammals evaluated and alternative processing of the preproMCH peptide can generate two additional putative peptides, designated neuropeptide E-I (NEI) and neuropeptide G-E (NGE) (Nahon et al., 1989). Several in vivo studies have shown that MCH plays a role in a variety of physiologic processes mediated within the central nervous system (CNS), including energy homeostasis sleep and arousal, and emotionality (Yumiko and Nagasaki, 2008; Torterolo et al., 2009). Although less studied, MCH may also have a role in peripheral tissues such as in gut and pancreatic islet function (Pissios et al., 2007; Kokkotou et al., 2008).

Two MCH G-protein coupled receptors (GPCRs) have been characterized (Pissios et al., 2006; Chung et al., 2011). MCHR1 is found in all vertebrates, while MCHR2 is found in non-rodent higher species, including primates (Hill et al., 2001; Sailer et al., 2001).

Neurobiology, rodent genetics, and rodent pharmacologic studies all demonstrate that MCH and the MCH receptors are involved in regulating body weight (Gomori et al., 2003, 2007; Hervieu, 2006; Bednarek, 2007; Antal-Zimanyi and Khawaja, 2009; Johansson, 2011; Cheon, 2012). On the basis of this information, many pharmaceutical companies have pursued the development of MCHR1 antagonists for the treatment of obesity (for a recent review, see Johansson, 2011). Unfortunately, although a few MCHR1 antagonists have entered development, no compound has successfully demonstrated anti-obesity efficacy in a clinical trial. It remains unclear if this lack of clinical efficacy is due to a lack of efficacy via the MCH1R pathway or to the inability of teams to identify safe and well-tolerated compounds with sufficient potency and pharmacodynamics properties to test the hypothesis. This review summarizes the evidence for a role of MCH and its receptors in energy homeostasis and the progress made to date toward identifying small-molecule antagonists to treat obesity.

Go to:

MCH Acts through Two G-Protein Coupled Receptors

Originally described as the orphan receptor SLC-1/GPR24 (Kolakowski et al., 1996), MCHR1 was later shown by five groups to be activated by MCH (Pissios et al., 2006). The 402-amino acid rodent and human MCHR1 receptors are highly homologous, sharing ~95% identity (Pissios and Maratos-Flier, 2003), and the highest expression of the receptors is within the brain (Saito et al., 1999; Hill et al., 2001). Like many family A GPCRs, the MCHR1 receptors have consensus N-glycosylation sites at the amino terminus and several potential phosphorylation sites in the intracellular loops (Lakaye et al., 1998).

In recombinant cell lines, the natural ligand, MCH, binds to MCHR1 with ~1 nM affinity, and it couples to Gi, Go, and Gq proteins (Hawes et al., 2000; Pissios et al., 2003). Thus, activation of MCHR1 leads to an increase in intracellular Ca++ accumulation acting through the Gq-coupled pathway and/or to lowered cyclic adenosine monophosphate (cAMP) levels via the Gi/o-coupled pathway. Further analyses of the signaling of MCHR1 in recombinant cell lines and in brain slices demonstrates that activation of MCHR1 also leads to ERK phosphorylation (Pissios et al., 2003). In 3T3-L1 adipocytes, MCH rapidly induced a threefold to fivefold increase in MAPK pathway activities (Bradley et al., 2002). It is unclear if all, or some, of these signaling pathways contribute to MCH-mediated events in vivo.

A second MCHR was later identified and termed MCHR2 by six groups (Antal-Zimanyi and Khawaja, 2009). The functional role of MCHR2 is not well defined, in part because it is not expressed in rodents and related species (hamsters, guinea pigs, or rabbits), but it is expressed in humans, dogs, ferrets, and monkeys (Tan et al., 2002). The amino acid sequence identity between MCHR1 and MCHR2 is low, ~38%, with the highest homology in the seven-transmembrane domains that form the ligand binding pocket (Sailer et al., 2001). Although MCH binds to MCHR1 and MCHR2 with a similar nanomolar affinity, the signal transduction mechanism of MCHR2 is limited to the Gq-mediated increase in intracellular Ca++ levels (Sailer et al., 2001). MCHR2 is largely co-expressed with MCHR1 in the CNS (Sailer et al., 2001), although peripheral expression was also found in adipocytes, pancreas, prostate, and intestine (An et al., 2001). The phylogenetic tree of MCH-related receptors contains opioid, somatostatin, galanin, urotensin 2, and orphan receptors (Sailer et al., 2001). MCH receptors have the highest homology (about 40%) with the somatostatin receptors (Sailer et al., 2001).

Go to:

Neuroanatomy of MCH and MCH Receptors

Melanin-concentrating hormone has been implicated in many behaviors. The hypothalamus is one of the primary sites in which MCH-containing nerve fibers and MCH receptors are extensively expressed (Gao, 2009). Although most of the MCH neurons are located within the incerto-hypothalamic and lateral hypothalamic area (LHA), a recent review by Bittencourt details the locations throughout the brain of MCH nerve terminals (Bittencourt, 2011). Neural signaling by MCH via its receptors has been implicated in the control of energy balance, but due to the wide distribution of MCH-containing fibers throughout the brain, the critical sites of action for particular behaviors have not been identified (Zheng et al., 2005). In male rats, neurons expressing MCH are found in the LHA and medial zona incerta, as well as, sparsely, in the olfactory tubercle and pontine reticular formation. The wide distribution of MCH fibers suggests the involvement of this neuropeptide in a variety of functions, including arousal, neuroendocrine control, and energy homeostasis (Rondini et al., 2007).

Melanin-concentrating hormone-expressing neurons in the LHA play an integrative role between signals from the periphery, acting via first-order neurons in the arcuate nucleus, and then from extra-hypothalamic systems, which modulate regulation of feeding, drinking, and seeking behaviors (Guyon et al., 2009). Factors from the periphery affect brain activity, resulting in changes in food intake and energy expenditure. Neurons from the arcuate nucleus detect changes in homeostatic parameters and transmit information to other brain areas, including the LHA. These secondary area neurons have widespread projections throughout the brain, and their activation leads to coordinated and altered behaviors (Guyon et al., 2009). About 25% of the LHA neurons projecting to the pedunculopontine tegmental (PPT) nucleus are immunoreactive for MCH, and 75% of the LHA neurons projecting to the cerebral motor cortex also contain MCH (Elias et al., 2008). Also, 15% of the incerto-hypothalamic neurons projecting to the PPT express MCH immunoreactivity. The MCH neurons express glutamic acid decarboxylase mRNA, a gamma-aminobutyric acid (GABA) synthesizing enzyme, indicating that the MCH/GABA neurons are involved in inhibitory modulation and their activation may lead to decreased motor activity in states of negative energy balance (Elias et al., 2008). Like MCH, vasopressin and oxytocin can influence energy homeostasis and other behaviors. Whole-cell recording in hypothalamic brain slices from the MCH-green fluorescent protein transgenic mouse revealed that both vasopressin and oxytocin evoked a substantial excitatory effect on MCH-expressing cells (Yao et al., 2012). Both neuropeptides reversibly increased spike frequency and depolarized the membrane potential in a concentration-dependent manner, suggesting that vasopressin or oxytocin exerts a robust excitatory effect on presumptive GABA cells that contain MCH (Yao et al., 2012).

Interestingly, projections to ventral medullary sites apparently play a role in the inhibitory effect of MCH on energy expenditure, but not food intake (Zheng et al., 2005). In the rat, a significant proportion (5–15%) of primarily perifornical and far-lateral hypothalamic MCH neurons project to the dorsal vagal complex. Retrograde tracing in the caudal brainstem demonstrated that MCH-immunoreactive axons are distributed densely in the nucleus of the solitary tract, in the dorsal motor nucleus of the vagus, and in sympathetic premotor areas in the ventral medulla (Zheng et al., 2005). In medulla slice preparations, MCH inhibited the amplitude of excitatory postsynaptic currents. Administration of MCH in the fourth ventricle in freely moving rats decreased core body temperature, but it did not change locomotor activity or food and water intake (Zheng et al., 2005).

The MCH pathways from the lateral hypothalamus to the mammillary nucleus may also enable the animal to look for food during the initial moments of appetite stimulation (Casatti et al., 2002). Injection of the retrograde tracer True Blue in the medial mammillary nucleus led to MCH/True Blue double-labeled neurons in the LHA, the rostromedial zona incerta, and the dorsal tuberomammillary nucleus. The afferents were confirmed using implants of the anterograde tracer Phaseolus vulgaris leucoagglutinin. The MCH projections may participate in spatial memory processing mediated by the medial mammillary nucleus (Casatti et al., 2002).

In addition to the LHA, the nucleus accumbens shell (AcSh) is a brain region important for food intake. The AcSh contains high levels of receptor for MCH. MCH receptor activation in the AcSh increases food intake, while AcSh MCH receptor blockade reduces feeding. Moreover, in vivo recordings confirm that MCH reduces neuronal activity in the AcSh in freely moving animals, consistent with a model from other pharmacological and electrophysiological studies whereby reduced AcSh neuronal firing leads to food intake (Sears et al., 2010). Since the AcSh mediates reinforcing properties of food, MCH may modulate motivational aspects of feeding. Indeed, chronic loss of rat MCH decreased food intake predominantly via a reduction in meal size during development and reduced high-fat food reinforced operant response in adult rats (Mul et al., 2011). Also, chronic loss of ProMCH in the rat affects the limbic dopamine system, since adult Pmch-/- rats showed increased ex vivo electrically evoked dopamine release (Mul et al., 2011). Thus, MCH actions in the AcSh mediate motivational aspects of feeding behavior.

MCHR1 is widely distributed in the brain (Hervieu et al., 2000; Able et al., 2009). Hervieu et al. (2000) used in situ hybridization histochemistry and immunohistochemistry to determine that Mchr1 mRNA and protein were widely expressed throughout the rat brain. Similar to the distribution of MCH, Mchr1 signals were observed in the cerebral cortex, caudate-putamen, hippocampal formation, amygdala, hypothalamus, and thalamus, as well as in various nuclei of the mesencephalon and rhombencephalon (Hervieu et al., 2000). Able et al. (2009) used an MCHR1-specific radioligand to demonstrate highly MCHR1-specific binding in the rat nucleus accumbens, caudate-putamen, and preform cortex, as well as lower levels of binding in the hippocampus and amygdala. Surprisingly, and in contrast to Hervieu et al. (2000) and Able et al. (2009) did not detect MCHR1 binding in the hypothalamus.

The distribution of MCHR2 in the primate brain nearly overlaps that of MCHR1, but the latter shows much higher relative levels and a wider distribution pattern (Mori et al., 2001). MCHR2 is expressed in several human brain areas, including the hippocampus and amygdala, although its distribution in the hypothalamus remains controversial. Specifically, MCHR2 mRNA was reported to be mainly expressed in the arcuate nucleus and ventromedial hypothalamic nucleus in African green monkeys by in situ hybridization (Sailer et al., 2001), while three other reports did not detect its expression in the human hypothalamus by RT-PCR (Hill et al., 2001; Mori et al., 2001) or Northern blot analysis (Rodriguez et al., 2001).

Go to:

Human Genetics of MCH and Energy Homeostasis

Genetic analysis of obese subjects has identified several variants of MCH and the MCH receptors, but no alterations have been conclusively linked to obesity or leanness. In an association study, among 106 subjects with severe early onset obesity and a history of hyperphagia, two missense variants were found in MCHR1: Y181H and R248Q (Gibson et al., 2004). Neither of these was found in 192 normal-weight controls. R248Q co-segregated with obesity across two generations, but family data were unavailable for Y181H. When tested for functional response, the R248Q variant showed no evidence of constitutive activation, alteration in cAMP signaling, or ligand hypersensitivity (Gibson et al., 2004). Two common single-nucleotide polymorphisms (SNPs) were found to be in linkage disequilibrium, but no association between either of these and obesity-related phenotypes was found among a population cohort of 541 whites. Only two rare, non-coding variants were found in MCHR2. However, the relationship of these MCHR2 variants to metabolic phenotypes has not been clarified (Gibson et al., 2004). Genomic screening of 13.4 kb encompassing the MCHR1 in extremely obese German children and adolescents identified 11 infrequent variations and two SNPs in the MCHR1 coding sequence and 18 SNPs (eight were novel) in the flanking sequence. Although an association of an MCHR1 haplotype (SNPs rs133072 and rs133073) with obesity was observed in two cohorts of German children and adolescents, it was not confirmed in five independent cohorts (Wermter et al., 2005). To investigate the possible polygenic role of MCHR1, six common SNPs (minor allele frequency >5%) found in the sequenced regions were screened in 557 morbidly obese adults, 552 obese children, and 1195 non-obese non-diabetic control subjects (Bell et al., 2005). The plausible promoter SNP, rs133068, was found to be associated with protection against obesity in obese children only (Bell et al., 2005).

A functional analysis of 11 MCHR1 variants that had been reported previously in the literature identified two mutant receptors, R210H and

P377S, that failed to respond to MCH (Goldstein et al., 2010). Five other variants showed significant alterations in MCH efficacy, ranging from 44 to 142% of the wild-type value. Both inactive receptors had cell surface expression that was comparable to wild-type (Goldstein et al., 2010). It is of note that the two loss-of-function mutants were identified in markedly underweight individuals, raising the possibility that a lean phenotype may be linked to deficient MCHR1 signaling (Goldstein et al., 2010). Additional association studies with larger cohorts are needed to explore the extent to which signaling-deficient MCHR1 variants influence the maintenance of body weight.

The association between MCHR2 variation and human obesity was investigated in 141 obese children and 24 non-obese adult subjects by DNA sequencing, and by case-control analyses using 628 severely obese children and 1401 controls (Ghoussaini et al., 2007). None of the MCHR2 variants showed an association with adult severe obesity, but the A76A SNP was associated with severe obesity (P = 0.01) and overeating in obese children (P = 0.02) (Ghoussaini et al., 2007). Validation of an association of MCHR2 with obesity requires replication in other cohorts.

The common allele of the ProMCH gene, rs7973796, may be associated with a higher body mass index (BMI) in olanzapine-treated patients with schizophrenia. In a subgroup of subjects under 50 years of age among 300 schizophrenia patients, the rs7973796 genotype was associated with an effect on BMI among patients taking olanzapine (interaction P = 0.025) (Chagnon et al., 2007). Olanzapine-treated patients with schizophrenia carrying the homozygote genotype showed a higher BMI for rs7973796 (P = 0.016 with the least-squares means t-test) than the variant homozygotes. The G allele was associated with an increase in the odds of obesity in schizophrenic patients taking olanzapine (Chagnon et al., 2007).

Go to:

Rodent Genetics Indicate a Role for MCH in Energy Homeostasis

Multiple mouse knockout (KO) models have been constructed to explore the role of MCH in energy homeostasis and other MCH-mediated behaviors. The KO models include multiple constructs that prevent synthesis of MCH and the MCHR1 receptor. Studies of these mice show that loss of MCH function leads to leanness and resistance to obesity.

MCH KO mice

Strong evidence that MCH mediates energy homeostasis came from studies of mice in which the Promch gene was inactivated. Mice constructed with targeted inactivation of the Promch gene in a mixed C57BL/6 × 129SvJ genetic background had reduced body weight and leanness due to hypophagia (reduced feeding) and an increased metabolic rate, despite reduced amounts of both leptin and arcuate nucleus proopiomelanocortin mRNA (Shimada et al., 1998). Evaluation of Promch inactivation in pure genetic backgrounds confirmed that Promch deficiency increased energy expenditure and promoted increased running-wheel activity (Kokkotou et al., 2005; Zhou et al., 2005). As observed previously on a mixed background, the C57BL/6 Promch KO mice were hypophagic; however, the 129SvEv Promch KOs were hyperphagic, relative to wild-type. In both C57BL/6 and 129SvEv backgrounds, deletion of Promch led to reduced adiposity, attenuated weight gain, and increased locomotor activity, compared with wild-type counterparts. The relative increase in activity was greater on a high-fat diet (HFD) than on regular chow (Kokkotou et al., 2005). The lean phenotype of the Promch KO mice persisted as the mice aged. At 19 months, C57BL/6 Promch-/- male and female mice weighed about 25% less than their wild-type counterparts as a result of reduced fat mass in Promch-/- mice. The aged Promch-/- mice exhibited improved glucose tolerance in intraperitoneal glucose tolerance tests, were more insulin sensitive, and were more active compared with wild-type controls (Jeon et al., 2006).

Further confirmation of the role of MCH in energy homeostasis came from studies of Promch neuron-ablated mice, generated using toxin (ataxin-3)-mediated ablation strategy in an FVB/n background (Alon and Friedman, 2006). In these mice, the Promch gene is present throughout development, but 60–70% of MCH-expressing neurons degenerate in the first few weeks of life (Alon and Friedman, 2006). After 7 weeks of age, the mice developed reduced body weight, body length, fat mass, lean mass, and leptin levels. As observed in the C57BL/6 Promch-/- mice, leanness was characterized by hypophagia and increased energy expenditure. In leptin-deficient ob/ob mice, loss of either Promch or MCH-containing neurons improved obesity, diabetes, and hepatic steatosis, suggesting that MCH is an important mediator of the response to leptin deficiency (Segal-Lieberman et al., 2003; Alon and Friedman, 2006).

Promch tg mice

The phenotype of Promch tg mice overexpressing MCH also supports a role for MCH in energy homeostasis. Ludwig et al. (2001) constructed transgenic mice that overexpressed Promch in the lateral hypothalamus at ~ twofold higher levels than normal mice. On an FVB background, the homozygous transgenic mice fed a HFD ate 10% more and were 12% heavier than wild-type animals. Blood glucose levels were higher both preprandially and after an intraperitoneal glucose injection, and the transgenic mice were insulin-resistant (Ludwig et al., 2001). Promch tg heterozygous mice on a C57Bl/6 background were hyperphagic on regular chow, heavier, and insulin-resistant, but did not have elevated blood glucose (Ludwig et al., 2001).

Mchr1-/- mice

As the gene for preproMCH encodes two additional peptides, NEI and NGE of unknown function (Nahon et al., 1989), studies with Mchr1 KO mice provided clarification and confirmation of the role of MCH in energy homeostasis. Three groups independently produced Mchr1-/- mice. Chen et al. (2002) reported that Mchr1 KO mice on a C57BL/6 × 129SvJ mixed background were resistant to diet-induced obesity and had fat mass that was significantly lower in both male (4.7 ± 0.6 vs. 9.6 ± 1.2 g) and female (3.9 ± 0.2 vs. 5.8 ± 0.5 g) mice than that of the wild-type control. The mice were hyperphagic on a HFD, but had a 28% higher metabolic rate than wild-type. Both leptin and insulin levels were significantly lower in male Mchr1-/- mice than in the wild-type controls, but there were no detectable differences in glucose levels. No differences were observed between heterozygotes and wild-type mice (Chen et al., 2002). Marsh et al. (2002) observed that Mchr1-/- mice also constructed on a C57BL/6 × 129SvJ mixed background had normal body weights, yet they had reduced fat mass and were hyperphagic when maintained on regular chow. In agreement with Chen et al. (2002) they observed that Mchr1-/- mice were less susceptible to diet-induced obesity, and the KO leanness was a consequence of hyperactivity and altered metabolism (Marsh et al., 2002). A later study by Zhou et al. (2005) showed that the Mchr1 KO mice had a dramatic 250% increase in running-wheel activity along with hyperphagia (Antal-Zimanyi and Khawaja, 2009). Astrand et al. (2004) also independently generated Mchr1-/- mice on a mixed C57BL/6 × 129SvJ background and observed that the mice had an elevated metabolic rate and were hyperactive, hyperphagic, and lean. A >12% increase in heart rate without any change in blood pressure was noted (Astrand et al., 2004). Two groups studied Mchr1 KO mice after backcrossing onto a C57BL/6 background (Bjursell et al., 2006; Ahnaou et al., 2011). In leptin-deficient ob/ob mice, loss of Mchr1 reduced adiposity (although body weights were not statistically different), improved the response in an oral glucose tolerance test (OGTT), increased spontaneous movement, and improved thermoregulation upon exposure to cold, suggesting that MCH is an important mediator of the response to leptin deficiency (Bjursell et al., 2006).

The role of MCHR2 has not been investigated in animal models. MCHR2 is absent in rodents but is present in higher species, including primates (Hill et al., 2001; Sailer et al., 2001). The role of MCHR2 might be studied in MCHR2-humanized mice, but no such model has been described. Alternatively, in vivo studies with MCHR1- and MCHR2-selective agonists could be used to study the role of MCHR2 in non-rodent species with a functional MCHR2. Indeed, it is surprising that in vivo pharmacological studies with selective ligands have not been performed, in light of the availability of MCH peptides that are potent dual MCHR1/R2 agonists, selective MCHR1 agonists, MCHR2-preferring agonists, and potent MCHR1/R2 antagonists (MacNeil and Bednarek, 2009). At this point, it is unclear if MCHR1 and MCHR2 play redundant or unique roles in MCH signaling in primates, or whether MCHR2 plays any significant role in energy homeostasis in humans.

Multiple mouse models show that disruption of the MCH system, via either the peptide ligand or the receptor, results in altered energy homeostasis (Table

(Table1).
1). In general, loss of MCH signaling leads to a lean, diet-induced obese (DIO)-resistant phenotype due primarily to increased energy expenditure, and in some models, lower food intake.

Table 1

Mouse genetic models supporting a role for MCH in energy homeostasis.

Genotype	Phenotype	Reference
Promch-/	Hypophagic, reduced	Shimada et al.

-C57BL/6 × 129SvJ	adiposity, increased metabolic rate, and reduced weight	(1998)
Promch-/- C57BL/6	Normophagic, reduced adiposity, increased activity and metabolic rate, and reduced weight	Zhou et al. (2005), Kokkotou et al. (2005)
Promch-/ -C57BL/6 × 129SvEv	Hyperphagic, reduced adiposity, increased activity and metabolic rate, and reduced weight	Kokkotou et al. (2005)
Promch;ataxin-3 FVB/n	Hypophagic, reduced adiposity, increased metabolic rate, normo-activity, and reduced weight	Alon and Friedman (2006)
Promch;ataxin-3; ob/ob (FVB/ nXC57BL/6)	Hyperphagic, reduced adiposity, reduced glucose, reduced steatosis, and reduced weight	Alon and Friedman (2006)
Promch-/-;ob/ob C57BL/6	Reduced adiposity, reduced glucose, increased metabolic rate, increased activity, and reduced weight	Segal-Lieberman et al. (2003)
Promch tg/tg FVB	Increased weight, hyperphagic on HFD, increased glucose, and insulin-resistant	Ludwig et al. (2001)
Promch tg/+ C57BL/6	Increased weight, hyperphagic on chow, normo-glucose, and insulin-resistant	Ludwig et al. (2001)
Mchr1-/ - C57BL/6 × 129SvJ	Reduced adiposity, hyperphagic, hyperactive, reduced weight, higher metabolic rate, and reduced insulin	Marsh et al. (2002), Chen et al. (2002), Astrand et al. (2004), Zhou et al. (2005)
Mchr1-/	No differences vs. wild-	Chen et al. (2002)

+ C57BL/6 × 129SvJ	type	
Mchr1 -/- C57BL/6	Reduced insulin, improved OGTT, and elevated body temperature	Bjursell et al. (2006), Ahnaou et al. (2011)
Mchr1 -/-;ob/ob C57BL/6	Decreased adiposity, reduced insulin, improved OGTT, increased activity	Bjursell et al. (2006)

Open in a separate window

Go to:

Pharmacologic Studies Confirm a Role for MCH in Energy Homeostasis

In vivo studies have shown that MCH or MCH analogs increase food intake and body weight, while, conversely, studies with MCHR1 antagonists reduce body weight and associated comorbidities.

In vivo effects of MCH peptide agonists

Melanin-concentrating hormone, and occasionally MCH derivatives, have been used to evaluate the role of MCH in energy homeostasis. Most studies have utilized acute injections of MCH into either specific brain nuclei or, more commonly, the third or fourth ventricle. These injections almost certainly lead to supraphysiologic levels of MCH in at least some of the MCH receptor-containing nuclei. Qu et al. (1996) were the first to show that intracerebroventricular (ICV) MCH increased food intake. In multiple experiments ICV injections of 5 or 30 µg into Long Evans rats increased 2-, 4-, and 6-h food intake between 150 and 200% (Qu et al., 1996). ICV injection of MCH into the third ventricle of either Wistar or Sprague-Dawley rats also increased food intake (Qu et al., 1996; Della-Zuana et al., 2002; Shearman et al., 2003). The orexigenic effects of ICV MCH were maximal at 2 h post injection (Della-Zuana et al., 2002). In Wistar rats, low doses (0.1 and 0.5 µg/rat) were ineffective, while higher doses (1, 5, and 10 µg/rat) were equally effective, leading to an approximate doubling of food intake over 2–4 h (Della-Zuana et al., 2002). In Sprague-Dawley rats, only the two highest doses led to significant increases in food intake (Della-Zuana et al., 2002). When presented with sucrose solutions after ICV injection of MCH (2 nmol), Sprague-Dawley rats increased their intake of sucrose solution by increasing the rate of licking (Baird et al., 2006). The role of MCH in energy homeostasis was also confirmed in sheep, which have both MCHR1 and MCHR2; acute

ICV doses of MCH increased food intake (Whitlock et al., 2005). Potent MCH analogs (IC50 < 25 nM), but not the weak analogs (IC50 > 1000 nM), reduced 2-h food intake after ICV administration of 4.4 nmol to Wistar rats (Suply et al., 2001). In a separate study in Sprague-Dawley rats using a smaller, potent MCH analog, Shearman et al. (2003) observed dose-dependent increases in 6-h food intake after an ICV injection of an MCH agonist (1 µg/rat, +68%; 5 µg/rat, +76%; 15 µg/rat, +122%). Guesdon et al. (2008) confirmed that the smaller MCH analog, when given ICV at 5 µg/rat, increased food intake in Wistar rats threefold over a 2-h period.

Intracerebroventricular injection of MCH into the third ventricle of rats significantly increased the ingestion of sucrose and glucose solution, but not of saccharin, indicating that the MCH-induced dipsogenic response is more related to caloric content than to sweet taste per se (Sakamaki et al., 2005). Injections of MCH into several brain nuclei led to increases in food intake. MCH (0.6 nmol) elicited a rapid and significant increase in feeding in satiated rats following injection into the arcuate nucleus, the paraventricular nucleus, or the dorsomedial nucleus (Abbott et al., 2003). However, no significant alteration in feeding was observed following injection into other brain regions associated with energy homeostasis, including the supraoptic nucleus, LHA, medial preoptic area, anterior hypothalamic area, or ventromedial nucleus of the hypothalamus (Abbott et al., 2003).

In a side-by-side comparison, MCH was found to be a weaker orexigen than two other hypothalamic neuropeptides. In lean rats, 1 and 3 nmol of the ICV-injected orexigenic peptides, neuropeptide Y (NPY) and agouti-related protein (AGRP), showed robust increases in intake of a sucrose solution, but 3 nmol of MCH mediated only a non-significant trend toward increased feeding (Semjonous et al., 2009). The importance of forebrain hypothalamic regions for MCH action was apparent when injection of 6 nmol of MCH into the fourth ventricle of lean rats or sheep failed to induce increased food intake, while control injections of NPY did increase food intake (Whitlock et al., 2005; Baird et al., 2007). Administration of LiCl, a potent inducer of conditioned taste aversion (CTA), to rats leads to an upregulation of Mch and Mchr1 mRNA (Mitra et al., 2012). However, when MCH was injected prior to the induction of CTA with LiCl, as well as later during the CTA retrieval, MCH treatment did not reduce the magnitude of CTA upon subsequent presentations of the aversive tastant (Mitra et al., 2012). Thus, MCH is not critical to the development of CTA.

Although most ICV studies leading to an increase in food intake utilized injection into the third ventricle, Georgescu et al. (2005) demonstrated that direct injection of 1 μg of MCH into the AcSh, a region rich in MCHR1, resulted in a robust increase in food intake by Sprague-Dawley rats lasting at least 4 h. Guesdon et al. (2008) used a potent, truncated MCH analog and also observed that injection of 5 μg into the AcSh of Wistar rats increased food intake of regular chow threefold during the 2 h following injection.

Agonist studies in preproMCH-deficient rats confirmed that the orexigenic actions of MCH are independent of two other preproMCH encoded peptides, NGE and NEI. Acute AcSh administration of NGE and NEI, or chronic ICV infusion of NEI, did not affect feeding behavior in adult Promch+/+ or Promch−/− rats (Mul et al., 2011). However, acute administration of MCH to the AcSh of adult Promch−/− rats elevated feeding behavior toward wild-type levels (Mul et al., 2011).

In addition to the effects of MCH on food intake, the role of MCH in mediating energy expenditure was also compared with that of two other orexigenic peptides, AGRP and orexin. Both AGRP and orexin, administered ICV (1 nmol/mouse), significantly decreased oxygen consumption compared with artificial cerebrospinal fluid (aCSF) treated controls; in contrast, MCH (1 nmol/mouse) had no significant effect compared with aCSF-treated controls (Asakawa et al., 2002). However, an effect of MCH on oxygen consumption might not have been detected, since only a relatively low dose of peptide was tested.

Chronic ICV infusions of MCH into rodents were shown to not only increase food intake, but to also cause obesity (Della-Zuana et al., 2002; Gomori et al., 2003; Ito et al., 2003); while MCH-induced insulin resistance in rats was observed acutely in the absence of weight changes (Pereira-da-Silva et al., 2005). Chronic infusions of MCH (8 μg/rat/day) over 12 days led to an increase in body weight of about 20 g more than did control aCSF infusions in both Wistar or Sprague-Dawley rats (Della-Zuana et al., 2002). After a 14-day infusion of MCH into the third ventricle of C57BL/6J mice (10 μg/day), no significant increase in food intake was observed in mice fed a regular chow, but on a moderately high-fat diet (MHF), the mice ate about 15% more food (Gomori et al., 2003). Mice on both diets were significantly heavier than control mice, with the largest increase in body weight observed in the MCH infused mice on a MHF diet;

these mice gained 17% more weight than the control infused mice on an MHF diet (Gomori et al., 2003). Glick et al. (2009) also observed that chronic infusion of 10 μg/day of MCH for 14 days into C57BL/6 mice fed regular chow led to a 34% increase in food intake and a 15% increase in body weight after a 14-day infusion. In a separate study, C57BL/6J mice on an MHF diet infused with a lower amount of MCH (3 μg/day for 7 days) also were hyperphagic and gained 350% more weight than did the vehicle control mice, with no detectable changes in activity (Ito et al., 2003). In addition, a small, potent, MCH analog given chronically ICV (30 μg/day) to Sprague-Dawley rats increased food intake by 23% and body weight by 38% more than in the vehicle controls (Shearman et al., 2003).

Intracerebroventricular-injected MCH has metabolic effects beyond increases in food intake and body weight. The acute effects of single MCH injections probably identify direct effects from increased MCH signaling in the brain, while the chronic effects may be subsequent to increased adiposity associated with body-weight gain. A single ICV injection of MCH into Wistar rats (3 nmol) inhibited the thyroid axis (Kennedy et al., 2001) by suppressing release of thyroid hormone from the hypothalamus, leading to a suppression of plasma thyroid-stimulating hormone (Kennedy et al., 2001). ICV injections of 4 nmol of MCH into Wistar rats for 4 days resulted in an ~ 10% increase in fasting plasma glucose (Pereira-da-Silva et al., 2005). Guesdon et al. (2008) used a potent, truncated MCH analog and found that injection of 5 μg into the AcSh or the third ventricle of Wistar rats did not significantly increase energy expenditure, but it did increase glucose oxidation and reduce lipid oxidation in the period 3 h after injection.

Chronic ICV infusions of MCH into C57BL/6J mice resulted in increased fat pad weights (~ 100%), leptin (~ 300%), liver triglycerides (~ 120%), fasting plasma glucose (~ 10%), and insulin (~ 100%) (Gomori et al., 2003). Glick et al. (2009) also observed that chronic infusion of 10 μg/ day of MCH for 14 days into C57BL/6 mice led to a 4.5-fold increase in adiposity, about a 0.4°C drop in body temperature during the active dark phase, a 15% decrease in oxygen utilization, and a 26% increase in plasma insulin-like growth factor 1 levels. Chronic MCH agonist infusions into Sprague-Dawley rats also led to increases in insulin (~ 200%) and leptin (~ 400%) (Shearman et al., 2003).

In vivo effects of MCH receptor antagonists

As discussed above, rodent genetic models clearly show a role for MCH in energy homeostasis. However, the applicability of these studies to understanding the physiological role and disease states associated with MCH signaling may be limited due to developmental effects of MCH inactivation or neuronal loss affecting other neuromodulators. Moreover, the relevance of in vivo pharmacology studies is complicated, because they utilize MCH and MCH agonists administered ICV at what are probably supraphysiologic levels. To better understand the role of MCH in energy homeostasis, a series of in vivo studies utilized MCHR1-specific antagonists. Because many pathways can affect food intake and body weight, in vivo effects of MCHR1 antagonists might be due to non-specific effects; however, in a few cases, researchers have demonstrated MCHR1 specificity by showing that an antagonist is inactive in Mchr1-/- mice.

Studies with MCHR1 peptidic antagonists Studies on truncated and substituted MCH analogs identified key amino acids for activation of the MCH receptors and led to synthesis of potent antagonist derivatives (Bednarek et al., 2002; Audinot et al., 2009). Several in vivo studies employed Ac-(Ava9–10, Ava14–15)-MCH(6–16)-NH2, a truncated, cyclic MCH analog containing γ-aminovaleric acid which is a potent (Kb 4 nM) antagonist (MacNeil and Bednarek, 2009). Shearman et al. (2003) reported that the peptide antagonist given ICV (10 µg) did not significantly reduce spontaneous feeding, affect feeding duration or locomotor activity, or alter overnight body-weight gain in lean male Sprague-Dawley rats. However, the peptide antagonist blocked the initial 2- or 3-h hyperphagic activity of an MCH agonist (Shearman et al., 2003; Mashiko et al., 2005). Chronic ICV infusion of the antagonist at 48 µg/day for 14 days reduced cumulative food intake by 13% and body-weight gain by 33%, relative to vehicle controls (Shearman et al., 2003). In male C57BL/6J mice fed an MHF diet, 28-day ICV infusion of the peptide antagonist at 7.5 µg/day decreased cumulative food intake 15% and the antagonist-treated mice weighed 13% less than the vehicle-infused controls (Mashiko et al., 2005). The antagonist treatment led to improvements in other metabolic parameters, including reductions in plasma glucose, leptin, insulin, and total cholesterol, as well as reductions in fat pad and liver weights (Mashiko et al., 2005). The specificity of the MCHR1 peptide antagonist was confirmed using Mchr1-/- mice, as infusion of the antagonist for 2 weeks had no effect on body weight, fat

mass, or cumulative food intake in the KO mice (Mashiko et al., 2005). In contrast to Mchr1 KO mouse models (Table
(Table1),
1), no changes were noted in activity after a 4-week infusion of the MCHR1 antagonist (Mashiko et al., 2005). Obese, aged, male C57BL/6J mice fed a HFD for 1 y (body weight ~ 60 g) were subjected to a 4-week ICV infusion with the peptide antagonist at 7.5 µg/day (Ito et al., 2008). The antagonist-infused mice lost 21% of their weight, while vehicle-infused mice gained 6% more weight. Not surprisingly, given the large differences in body weight, the MCHR1 antagonist-treated mice showed significant reductions in serum leptin and insulin (Ito et al., 2008). Also, the liver weights of the antagonist-treated DIO mice decreased by about 50%, while the serum liver markers showed improvements (Ito et al., 2008). In a follow-up study to explore the role of MCH in modulating accumulation of triglycerides in liver, male C57BL/6J mice were fed a diet deficient in methionine and choline to induce steatohepatitis; ICV treatment with the MCHR1 antagonist (7.5 µg/day for 10 days) did not result in any body-weight difference vs. vehicle control, but accumulation of triglycerides in liver was reduced 33% (Ito et al., 2008). The ability of MCHR1 antagonist treatment to improve hepatic steatosis was confirmed in a female model of obesity in which ovariectomized mice were fed a regular chow diet. Thirty weeks after the ovariectomy, the female C57BL/6J mice weighed about 25% more than did the sham treated mice (Gomori et al., 2007). When these obese mice were treated ICV with the MCHR1 peptide antagonist for 4 weeks at 7.5 µg/day, they lost 13% of their body weight and 32% of their liver triglycerides (Gomori et al., 2007).
Studies with S38151 in multiple rodent models of obesity resulted in significant effects on food intake and body weight. S38151 [p-guanidinobenzoyl-[des-Gly10]-MCH(7–17)] is a modified and truncated 11-amino acid MCH analog which is a potent (Kb = 4 nM) MCHR1 antagonist (Audinot et al., 2009). Injection of this peptidic MCHR1 antagonist into the AcSh reduced food intake (Georgescu et al., 2005). Over a 6-h period, in male Wistar rats, S38151 administered ICV dose dependently inhibited the orexigenic effects of previously injected MCH (Audinot et al., 2009). The highest doses of S38151, 30 and 50 nmol per rat, completely blocked MCH-induced food intake for 6 h (Audinot et al., 2009). The orexigenic effect of proMCH (131–165), which is more potent than MCH in stimulating feeding, was blocked for 2 h by 50 nmol/kg of S38151 administered ICV (Maulon-Feraille et al., 2002; Della-Zuana et al., 2012). Once daily ICV injections of 20 nmol/kg of S38151 into male Zucker fa/fa rats, reduced food intake,

water intake, motility, and body weight (Della-Zuana et al., 2012). A single injection of 20 µmol/kg of S38151 intraperitoneally (i.p.), reduced cumulative food intake in Zucker fa/fa rats for 24 h (Della-Zuana et al., 2012). S38151 was administered i.p. at 30 mg/kg for 5 days into two mouse models of obesity, female ob/ob and female C57BL/6J DIO mice, resulting in reductions in body weight and cumulative food intake. The S38151 effects on energy homeostasis were MCH1R based, since no changes in food intake or body weight were observed after 5 days of i.p. injection into female Mchr1 KO mice (Della-Zuana et al., 2012).

Studies with non-peptide MCHR1 antagonists The overwhelming set of genetic and physiologic data demonstrating that MCHR1 modulates energy homeostasis attracted the interest of a many medicinal chemistry groups who have synthesized numerous structurally distinct MCHR1 antagonists (see a recent review by Cheon, 2012). In all, 23 different companies have published more than 100 medicinal chemistry papers and patents describing attempts to optimize MCHR1 antagonist hit compounds toward drug candidates (see the recent review of the patent literature by Johansson, 2011). Many of the resulting optimized lead compounds, representing a diverse set of non-peptide MCHR1 antagonists, have been evaluated in vivo. Non-peptide MCHR1 antagonists are effective in different models of acute food intake in a variety of different rodent strains (Table
(Table2)
2) (Borowsky et al., 2002; Takekawa et al., 2002; Huang et al., 2005; Palani et al., 2005; McBriar et al., 2006; Sasikumar et al., 2006; Xu et al., 2006; Balavoine et al., 2007; Kowalski and Sasikumar, 2007; Moriya et al., 2009; Nagasaki et al., 2009; Haga et al., 2011; Kamata et al., 2011; Kasai et al., 2011, 2012). In general, MCHR1 antagonists potently block up to 75% of MCH-induced food intake (Borowsky et al., 2002; Takekawa et al., 2002; Moriya et al., 2009; Nagasaki et al., 2009), but they have more modest effects on reducing fasting-induced feeding and spontaneous feeding.

Table 2

Acute effects of non-peptide MCH1R antagonists on food intake.

Feeding model*	Time of measurement			Reference
	2 h	4, 5, or 6 h	24 h	

MCH-INDUCED HYPERPHAGIA IN RAT				
Male Sprague-Dawley		-90%		Takekawa et al. (2002)
Male Sprague-Dawley	-72%			Moriya et al. (2009)
Male Sprague-Dawley	-75%	-75%		Nagasaki et al. (2009)
Male Wistar	-70%			Borowsky et al. (2002)
FASTING-INDUCED FEEDING				
Male Wistar rats	-35%	-30%	-25%	Huang et al. (2005)
Mice (strain and gender unknown)	-80%	-40%		Balavoine et al. (2007)
DIO male C57BL/6NCrl:BR mice	-35%	-32%	-22%	McBriar et al. (2006)
DIO mice (strain and gender unknown)		-17%	-14%	Palani et al. (2005)
DIO mice (strain and gender unknown)	-12%	-20%	-9%	Sasikumar et al. (2006)
SPONTANEOUS FEEDING				
Male Sprague-Dawley rats			-30%	Kamata et al. (2011)
Female KK*Ay* mice	-63%			Kamata et al. (2011)
DIO C57BL/6J mice (gender unknown)			-19%	Haga et al. (2011)
DIO mice (strain and gender unknown)			-21%	Xu et al. (2006)
DIO male F344/Jcl rats			-30%	Kasai et al. (2012)
DIO male F344/Jcl rats		-28%		Kasai et al. (2011)

			-31%	Kowalski and Sasikumar (2007)
DIO male Sprague-Dawley rats			-31%	Kowalski and Sasikumar (2007)
Male Sprague-Dawley rats, ingestion of condensed milk#	-45%			Borowsky et al. (2002)

Open in a separate window

Data shown for the most potent analog in the cited reference at the highest dose tested. #Measured at 20 min.

Multiple MCHR1 antagonists have also shown dose-dependent and sustained efficacy in chronic models of obesity (Kym et al., 2005; Souers et al., 2005a,b, 2007; Vasudevan et al., 2005a,b; Carpenter et al., 2006; Hertzog et al., 2006; Tavares et al., 2006a,b; Mendez-Andino and Wos, 2007; Mendez-Andino et al., 2007; Gehlert et al., 2009; Ito et al., 2009; Semple et al., 2009; Suzuki et al., 2009; Hadden et al., 2010; Mihalic et al., 2012; Sasmal et al., 2012a,b). At the highest dose tested in DIO mice, ranging from 10 to 100 mpk, weight loss ranged from 5% at 5 days to 33% at 238 days (Ito et al., 2009; Mihalic et al., 2012). In several cases, weight loss was shown to be primarily due to the loss of fat mass (Souers et al., 2005a,b, 2007; Vasudevan et al., 2005a; Mendez-Andino et al., 2007). The mechanism of weight loss appears to involve a combination of reduced food intake, which was observed in six studies (Table

(Table3),
3), and increased energy expenditure with no increase in activity (Kowalski et al., 2006; Gehlert et al., 2009).

Table 3

Chronic effects of non-peptide MCH1R antagonists in rodents.

Rodent model of energy homeostasis*		
	Reduced food intake vs. vehicle (%)	Time (days)	Reference

REDUCED CUMULATIVE FOOD INTAKE IN MICE			
Male DIO C57BL/6J	16	5	Ito et al. (2009)
DIO (strain and gender unknown)	11	10	Mendez-Andino et al. (2007)
DIO (strain and gender unknown)	37	13	Kym et al. (2005)
DIO (strain and gender unknown)	13	14	Souers et al. (2005b)
Male DIO C57BL/6NCrl:BR	18	28	Kowalski et al. (2006)
REDUCED CUMULATIVE FOOD INTAKE IN RATS			
DIO Long Evans (gender unknown)	16	14	Gehlert et al. (2009)

	Weight loss vs. vehicle (%)	Time (days)	Reference
REDUCED BODY WEIGHT IN MICE			
DIO C57BL/6J male	5	5	Ito et al. (2009)
DIO C57BL/6J male	6	5	Surman et al. (2010)
DIO C57BL/6J male	6	6	Hadden et al. (2010)
DIO (strain and gender unknown)	8	7	Mendez-Andino and Wos (2007)
DIO (strain and gender unknown)	5	10	Mendez-Andino et al. (2007)
DIO AKR/J (gender unknown)	13	12	Hertzog et al. (2006)
DIO (strain and gender unknown)	18	13	Kym et al. (2005)
DIO C57BL/6J male	8	13	Suzuki et al. (2009)
DIO C57BL/6J	6	14	Vasudevan et al.

(gender unknown)			(2005b)
DIO C57BL/6J (gender unknown)	12	14	Sasmal et al. (2012a)
DIO C57BL/6J (gender unknown)	13	14	Sasmal et al. (2012b)
DIO (strain and gender unknown)	7	14	Souers et al. (2007)
DIO (strain and gender unknown)	23	14	Vasudevan et al. (2005a)
DIO (strain and gender unknown)	15	14	Souers et al. (2005a)
DIO (strain and gender unknown)	17	14	Souers et al. (2005b)
DIO AKR/J (gender unknown)	10	15	Carpenter et al. (2006)
DIO AKR/J (gender unknown)	10	21	Tavares et al. (2006b)
DIO AKR/J (gender unknown)	15	26	Tavares et al. (2006a)
DIO (strain and gender unknown)	31	28	Kym et al. (2005)
DIO C57BL/6NCrl:BR male	16	28	Kowalski et al. (2006)
DIO C57BL/6J (gender unknown)	9	137	Mihalic et al. (2012)
DIO female (strain unknown)	33	238	Mihalic et al. (2012)
REDUCED BODY WEIGHT IN RATS			
DIO Long Evans (gender unknown)	15	14	Gehlert et al. (2009)
DIO Sprague-Dawley male	15	14	Dyck et al. (2006)
DIO Wistar female	17	28	Semple et al. (2009)

Open in a separate window
Data shown for the most potent analog in the cited reference at the highest dose tested.
As shown above with peptides, and in Tables

Tables2
2 and

and3
3 with non-peptide compounds, many different MCHR1 antagonists have demonstrated modest to robust efficacy in a variety of rodent obesity models, suggesting that MCHR1 antagonists may have potential for treating human obesity. One caveat for the data is that in most cases, the antagonists have not demonstrated the ability to induce weight loss through an MCHR1-specific mode of action, since efficacy in *Mchr1* KO mice has not been evaluated. In fact, in one report of robust weight loss, the authors caution that some weight loss at the highest dose tested maybe due to non-specific mechanisms, since the compound resulted in high brain levels, 6.46 µg/g (Kym et al., 2005). However, in four reports, the MCHR1-specific efficacy of antagonists was confirmed, since the antagonists lacked efficacy in DIO *Mchr1* KO mice, but they showed body-weight loss in DIO wild-type mice (Gehlert et al., 2009; Della-Zuana et al., 2012; Mashiko et al., 2005; Mihalic et al., 2012). Further support for an MCHR1 mechanism based-weight loss has been reported for three compounds, for which efficacy was correlated with brain MCHR1 receptor occupancy (Hervieu et al., 2003; Kowalski et al., 2006; Ito et al., 2009).

Studies with MCHR2 antagonists The absence of the *Mchr2* in rodents has limited the interest in developing MCHR2-selective compounds. Only one paper has disclosed a potent MCHR2-selective non-peptide small-molecule antagonist (Chen et al., 2012). Compound 38 is a potent (Ki 13 nM) and selective MCHR2 antagonist with good oral bioavailability and pharmacokinetics suitable for *in vivo* studies (Chen et al., 2012). However, no *in vivo* data have been reported with this compound.

Clinical studies with MCHR1 antagonists

The intense interest in MCHR1 antagonists has resulted in more than 80 publications and 100 patent applications describing various unique antagonists (Johansson, 2011). Five compounds have reached testing in human subjects, but none has proceeded into advanced Phase II studies to rigorously test their efficacy in causing chronic weight loss (Figure

(Figure2).
2). A major issue with many lead compounds is increased cardiovascular risk due to high-affinity hERG binding and drug-induced QTc prolongation (Mendez-Andino and Wos, 2007).

The Amgen MCHR1 antagonist AMG 076 entered Phase I safety and tolerability testing in 2004, but there have been no subsequent reports of its status since 2005. GlaxoSmithKline MCHR1 antagonist GW-856464 also entered Phase I studies in 2004 (Cheon, 2012). However, on August 24, 2010, Carmen Drahl reported via Twitter that "low bioavailability precluded further development."

NGD-4715 is a selective MCHR1 antagonist developed by Neurogen. In a May 2, 2007 press release, Neurogen announced that NGD-4715 was safe and well-tolerated in a Phase I clinical trial. Neurogen was acquired by Ligand Pharmaceuticals in 2009; as of February 22, 2013, the Wikipedia entry for NGD-4715 quotes an e-mail from Ligand that there are "no plans for further development on the compound." In a May 31, 2011 press release, AMRI announced that its MCHR1 antagonist, ALB-127158(a), was well-tolerated in a Phase I single ascending-dose study and 14-

day multiple ascending-dose safety and tolerability study. An encouraging result reported by some subjects was loss of appetite. Despite the reported tolerability and suggestion of efficacy, in a subsequent press release dated October 4, 2011, AMRI announced that development was terminated before the initiation of Phase II studies.

Bristol–Myers Squibb (BMS) conducted the longest clinical trial with an MCHR1 antagonist. As of February 22, 2013, the BMS website indicates BMS-830216 was evaluated in a 28-day Phase I study to assess the safety, tolerability, and effect on body weight and other obesity-related factors of different doses of BMS-830216. A summary of the clinical results with BMS-830216 is available on the NIH website (http://www.ncats.nih.gov/files/BMS-830216.pdf), which indicates that BMS-830216 is a prodrug of the antagonist BMS-819881 and a potent ($K_i = 10\,nM$) and selective MCHR1 antagonist. BMS-830216 was generally safe and well-tolerated at all doses in the Phase I study for up to 28 days. However, no indications of weight loss or reduced food intake were observed, and the compound did not proceed to Phase II studies.

Go to:

Future Prospects

A rich literature of rodent genetics and rodent pharmacology demonstrates a significant role for MCH, acting via the MCHR1 within the hypothalamus, in maintaining energy homeostasis. This knowledge has stimulated more than 20 companies to seek MCHR1 selective compounds for the treatment of obesity. Five companies are known to have succeeded in identifying development candidates that proceeded through preclinical safety studies and enabled Phase I clinical safety and tolerability testing. Three of the compounds, NGD-4715, ALB-127158(a), and BMS-830216 (Figure

(Figure1),

1), were found generally safe and well-tolerated in the Phase I studies. However, BMS-830216, which was tested for 28 days in obese subjects, failed to show any significant weight loss efficacy. No compounds have proceeded into Phase II studies in which chronic efficacy could be evaluated.

After almost 15 years of research, studies have failed to detect anti-obesity efficacy with MCHR1 antagonists in the clinic. There are multiple reasons that might account for this disconnect between rodent and human studies. First, compounds tested in the clinic may not have had the appropriate properties to sufficiently block the MCHR1 receptor and achieve an effect of energy balance. For instance, the MCHR1 antagonists may not have reached the hypothalamic sites of MCH action. Since there have been no reported studies measuring the level of receptor occupancy of the clinical compounds, it is possible that the compounds failed to sufficiently penetrate the brain: blood barrier resulting in low and insufficient receptor occupancy. Second, studies utilizing a positron emission tomography (PET) ligand demonstrated that an NPY5R antagonist must achieve >90% receptor occupancy sustained over 24 h to cause weight loss (Erondu et al., 2006). Similarly, in DIO mouse studies, maximum weight loss was observed only when an MCHR1 antagonist blocked >90% of the MCHR1 receptors for 24 h (unpublished data by the author). Clearly, a MCHR1 PET ligand could guide compound dose selection to assure 24 h of high receptor blockade (Erondu et al., 2006; Philippe et al., 2012). Third, since humans also express MCHR2 in the hypothalamus (Sailer et al., 2001), MCH signaling in humans may involve both MCHR1 and MCHR2, such that blockade of the MCHR1 alone may not be sufficient to achieve efficacy in obesity. Fourth, the role of MCH in human energy homeostasis may not be as significant as its role in rodents, consequently, blockade of MCHR1 would be inherently ineffective as a treatment for obesity.

In the author's opinion, there is, at best, only a modest probability that an MCHR1 antagonist will be developed as a treatment for obesity. Following the failure of five Phase I compounds to progress to Phase II efficacy studies, the enthusiasm for MCHR1 antagonists has clearly dimmed. Moreover, after more than a decade of drug discovery effort by more than 20 companies, there are currently no known MCHR1 antagonists in the clinic for obesity. Should any company continue to seek MCHR1 antagonists, the author suggests that they should proceed only with the aid of a PET ligand, perhaps [11C]SNAP-7941, or another on-target biomarker to assess receptor occupancy (Philippe et al., 2012). Companies might also consider focusing their chemistry efforts on identifying a dual MCHR1 and MCHR2 antagonist, to assure that all MCH-mediated signaling involved in energy homeostasis is effectively blocked. Finally, an effective MCH antagonist therapy for obesity must not only achieve meaningful weight loss, but it must also be well-tolerated. Although not discussed in this review, there is significant rodent genetic and pharmacologic data indicating that MCH participates in other CNS behaviors (Saito and Nagasaki, 2008; Yumiko and Nagasaki, 2008; Antal-Zimanyi and Khawaja, 2009; Torterolo et al., 2009; Chung et al., 2011). In particular, studies in multiple rodent models suggest blockade of MCH signaling may be anxiolytic (Antal-Zimanyi and Khawaja, 2009; Chung et al., 2011). Tolerability may be a substantial hurdle for an effective MCH receptor antagonist to overcome.

The biggest problems that "Blackfolks" have is Obesity and Diabetes. Race Hustlers like Reginald would like you to believe that it's "Whitefolks"! No! In the Information Age or Education Age the biggest problem anyone could have is to be **UNEDUCATED**. Information is only good to the informed (educated). This also identifies anyone that would stand in your way of becoming informed as the BIGGEST OPPOSITION OR THE DEVIL!

You got some Nerve!!!

God (the Sun) speaks (emits radio waves) that you hear (absorb and convert) through your antenna (**the spine**). The nerves help distribute this information to the Plasma based Crystal disc, fitted with integrated circuits as well as gates and channels.

How can the eye of Heru and the Djed Pillar be so well known and yet I get attacked for discovering that the Was Scepter is the Aorta?

NEUROPATHY

Neuropathy - disease or dysfunction of one or more **peripheral nerves**, typically causing numbness or weakness. There are too may illnesses link to "bad nerves" to list or go through, in fact every aspect of your body is nerve dependent!

To be clear...

Peripheral Nervous System - The PNS consists of nerves and ganglia, which lie outside the brain and the spinal cord. The main function of the PNS is to connect the CNS to the limbs and organs, essentially serving as a relay between the brain and spinal cord and the rest of the body. **Unlike the CNS, the PNS is not protected by the vertebral column and skull, or by the blood–brain barrier, which leaves it exposed to toxins**.

The PNS is not just exposed to toxins, it is exposed to everything. This is why these nerves atrophy easily, especially without exercise.

*When the nerves attached to muscles fade, so to does strength, speed and hand-eye coordination.

*When the nerves attached to the adipocytes (fat cells) fade, so to does the ability to metabolize their contents. The crazy part is, even when the fat cells can't empty, THEY CAN STILL GET FATTER!!!

Sugar, estrogens, bacteria, toxins and viruses load up the fat cells, **FOR TEMPORARY STORAGE**. A broken nervous system stops the body from being able to clear this cargo. Nerve atrophy is just one more reason why its not just "diet and lifestyle".

The over simplification is based on ignorance and even worse an attempt to keep you ignorant. The moment you become more knowledgeable than your trainer, nutritionist, herbalist or doctor... they are fired and **they know it**!!! You are learning more than most of these guys have even been exposed to to earn their degrees or certifications, in fact after you read your 20th book from Dr. EnQi I want you to begin writing your book!

You didn't know it, but the Divine Mathematics Book and the AlgaRhythm Book, are your start! If you properly use those books, half of your first book will be written for you!!! In fact if you add your journey with the information and then the research from the books, **YOUR FIRST BOOK IS COMPLETE**!

YOU NEED TO BECOME TEACHERS! YOUR CREDENTIALS WILL BE YOUR BOOKS!

Cheat Codes - remember to research each cheat code in these books by cross referencing your goals or situation.

Calcium - Nerve Signalling

Copper - Ceruloplasmin, Dopamine-β-Hydroxylase, Macroglobulins, Copper/zinc Superoxide Dismutase, Cytochrome C Oxidase, Peptidylglycine A-Amidating Monooxygenase, Hephaestin and Lysyl Oxidase & all Cuproenzymes, Copper is required for actual Nerve Cell Development

EFA/Cholesterol - Protection of Nerve Cells

Chromium - Indirect action via Sugar Regulation

Magnesium - Every aspect of Nerve Function

B1 - Glucose Master Vitamin

B3 - NAD for the EnQi Cycle & the Sirtuin 7

B6 - Neurotransmitters

B12/Cobalt - Allows Metal Metabolism which is the foundation of the Nervous System, conversion of L-Methylmalonyl Coenzyme A into Succinyl Coenzyme A which is essential for formation of the Myelin Sheath

Thymoquinone - Nerve conduction, Velocity, Reduced Morphological Changes and Demyelination of the Sciatic Nerve

Vit D - Regulates Seratonin Release/Nerve Synthesis

Silver/Selenium/Zinc - Protection from Bugs/Oxidative Stress

Sodium/Potassium - Electrical Charge

Vit K - Sphingolipids (Neuron/Glial Cell Membranes) & Y-Glutamyl Carboxylase (formation of VKDPs & Gas6)

Chondrus Crispus

If you are suffering from a illness you may need emergency **CHOLESTEROL**! ESPECIALLY IF YOU HAVE BEEN ON A PLANT BASED DIET!

Coconut Meat or Eggs - Cholesterol

Curcumin - Schwann Cell recruitment, Myeline Regrowth & Neurogenesis (Nerve Regeneration)

You got some Nerve!!!

God (the Sun) speaks (emits radio waves) that you hear (absorb and convert) through your antenna (**the spine**). The nerves help distribute this information to the Plasma based Crystal disc, fitted with integrated circuits as well as gates and channels.

How can the eye of Heru and the Djed Pillar be so well known and yet I get attacked for discovering that the Was Scepter is the Aorta?

HUMAN ENGINEERING

Electronics is a scientific and engineering discipline that studies and applies the principles of physics to design, create, and operate devices that manipulate electrons and other electrically charged particles. Electronics is a subfield of electrical engineering which uses active devices such as **transistors, diodes, and integrated circuits** to control and amplify the flow of electric current and to convert it from one form to another, such as from alternating current (AC) to direct current (DC) or from analog signals to digital signals. - wiki

God (the Sun) speaks (emits radio waves) that you hear (absorb and convert) through your antenna (**the spine**). The nerves help distribute this information to the Plasma based Crystal disc, fitted with integrated circuits as well as gates and channels.

How can the eye of Heru and the Djed Pillar be so well known and yet I get attacked for discovering that the Was Scepter is the Aorta?

The trillions of Computer Chips you have in your Electronic Body are wired by these nerves. How is it possible that the spine is known by Kemetic Scientist and not it's make up? The spine is the **Motherboard**, I almost labeled it a backplane.

The difference is the connection to the waveguide we detail in the Movement book so we won't bore you with those details here... The spine not only is the hub for all the electrical wiring it produces blood!

We need to take another moment to discuss magic here. Nerves & Neurons literally convert electricity into chemistry. I mean your school textbooks say that electric from the axon is converted into chemicals in the synapse. In Melanin vs Diabetes book 1 we discuss the binary coding base for thought. In the Movement book we discuss the relationship of Emotions to Biochemistry. In the AlgaRhythm book we discuss the

Operating System that runs these programs for you "subconsciously". In the Fiscal Edition & L'Goat book (Melanocyte Gossip), we discuss the language of Cells.

Throughout all of these books we have discussed the EnQi Cycle and Pigment, this book is primarily dedicated to wiring and connection.

Atoms bond in a variety of ways however, the type of bonding determine how electrons and photons behave. In living crystal systems, complexity is based on the highest order of photons and electrons. This is why your bones and DNA are piezoelectric. This is why there is spontaneous chemiluminescence in your breath. Pigment in and throughout your body. All of the structures in your body are either Insulators (fat) or some type of conductors, for simplicity. The wiring connects all of these systems. You have Nerve and Neuron Systems and you have Circulatory Systems.

Modern External technology uses Coppering Wiring (electrons) or Fiber Optics (photons), the same way you do. You just have Nerves/Neurons (electric) and Pigments (photons).

When an electric wire comes in contact with information/power, there is a vibration or movement of electric charge or electrons in and around the wire. The charge flowing through and around the wire is known as the current. The Axon & Dendrites in a Nerve/Neuron are very high tech wiring.

Wires use different voltages to communicate via binary coding. Nerves/Neurons use high frequencies and low frequencies to release different molecules.

The Blood connects to the body's main processor (the brain) the aorta. Arterial pulsation regulates the flow of CSF.

Even the Breath is either a 1 or 0, inhale or exhale, CO_2 or Oxygen etc…

In the brain 10x as much blood is sent to the area of "thoth", than is required to power the "thinking". This is the root of system coupling, Arterial Pulse (& CSF), Nerve/Neuron activity and Blood itself.

CSF is produced by specialised ependymal cells in the choroid plexus of the ventricles of the brain, and absorbed in the arachnoid granulations. CSF occupies the subarachnoid space (between the arachnoid mater and the pia mater) and the ventricular system around and inside the brain and spinal cord. It fills the ventricles of the brain, cisterns, and sulci, as well as the central canal of the spinal cord. There is also a connection from the subarachnoid space to the bony labyrinth of the inner ear via the perilymphatic duct where the perilymph is continuous with the cerebrospinal fluid. The ependymal cells of the choroid plexus have multiple motile cilia on their apical surfaces that beat to move the CSF through the ventricles.

The choroid plexus consists of modified ependymal cells surrounding a core of capillaries and loose connective tissue. There is a choroid plexus in each of the four ventricles. In the lateral ventricles, it is found in the body, and continued in an enlarged amount in the atrium. There is no choroid plexus in the anterior horn. In the third ventricle, there is a small amount in the roof that is continuous with that in the body, via the interventricular foramina, the channels that connect the lateral ventricles with the third ventricle. A choroid plexus is in part of the roof of the fourth ventricle.

Unlike the ependyma, the choroid plexus epithelial layer has tight junctions[8] between the cells on the side facing the ventricle (apical surface). These tight junctions prevent the majority of substances from crossing the cell layer into the cerebrospinal fluid (CSF); thus the choroid plexus acts as a blood–CSF barrier. The choroid plexus folds into many villi around each capillary, creating frond-like processes that project into the ventricles. The villi, along with a brush border of microvilli, greatly increase the surface area of the choroid plexus. **CSF is formed as plasma is filtered from the blood through the epithelial cells**. Choroid plexus epithelial cells actively transport **sodium ions** into the ventricles and water follows the resulting osmotic gradient.

-    wiki

The Brain Cheat Codes:

Regulate/Avoid Histamine Gluten & Glutamate
Get large Amounts of EFAs & Healthy Cholesterol (Living Carbon)!!!

Selenium, Cysteine, Glutamine & Tryptophan - formulation of Glutathione Peroxidase lack of which leads to Uric Acid Recycling

Copper - Enzyme & Pigment Center Health

B Vitamins/Phosphorus/Nickel - Nutrient Metabolism

Gallium - Cellular Organization

Molybdenum/Manganese - Xanthine/Aldehyde/Sulfite Oxidase
(breakdown Uric Acid, Sulfur & Nitrogen Compounds)

Lithium/Rubidium - Brain Chemistry

Vit K - Boost Enzyme Function, Sphingolipid Production/Function
Hydration

Magnesium - Neuron Production/Ptrotection,
Glial Cells & Astrocyte Function

Plant Pigments

Natural Light in the Eyes

Limit Synthetic Light especially Blue

Aneurysm & Stroke Cheat Codes:

Copper/Vit C - enzyme lysyl oxidase (Potassium Cofactor)

Copper/Zinc - Superoxide Dismutase

Manganese - Superoxide Dismutase, Oxygen Liberation

B Vitamins - Iron Metabolism

EFAs - Tissue Pliability

Selenium - Prevents Lipid Oxidation which prevents
WBC build up and conversion into Foam Cells

Vit E - Reduce LDL levels

Calcium/EFAs/Resveratrol - Inhibits Clot Formation

Plant Pigments - Inhibit Fat Deposits

Gold - Foam Cell Inhibition

Vit C/Copper - Vessel Health

Iron/Copper - Electron/Oxygen Chain (nickel/cobalt cofactors)
B Vitamins - Nutrient Metabolism (phosphorus cofactor)

Germanium - WBC regulation

Porphyrins are Light Absorbers & Carriers. Heme (RBC & Mitochondria) absorb UV & Infrared Radiation. **DHA** converts photons into electrons in cells & tissues. The inner wall of Arteries, Veins & Capillaries are coated with **Glycoproteins**. The inner walls of Health "blood tunnels" should have a negative charge to match the negative charge of healthy RBCs. When like charges meet they repel one another this is how RBCs which are actually larger than capillaries, manage to fit through them. Loss of charge therefore causes blood clots!!!! Not too much **Vitamin K**!!!!! Keep in mind **Iron** Magnetizes minerals and pulls them through circulation so no iron no minerals circulation!!!!

Magnesium - maintains vascular pliability...

You got some Nerve!!!

God (the Sun) speaks (emits radio waves) that you hear (absorb and convert) through your antenna (**the spine**). The nerves help distribute this information to the Plasma based Crystal disc, fitted with integrated circuits as well as gates and channels.

How can the eye of Heru and the Djed Pillar be so well known and yet I get attacked for discovering that the Was Scepter is the Aorta?

ENQI'S TOTEM

The Reproductive System, The Spine and the Ventricles are all tied together by the Aorta. The Dr. EnQi Totem, Ankh, Was, Djed, Nekhbet & Shen, Eye of Heru & the Naga. We have decoded these as the Reproductive System symbolic of Electromagnetism (male/female), the Aorta, the Spine, Rebirth & HGT (cross species and family line "pollination" of the brain), the Brain & 3rd Ventricle (info processing). When you look at the following info graphic I have created, notice the 7x Thoth.

7x Thoth = Knowledge = Light = God

Can you explain to me HOW "KEMETIC SCHOLARS" make the claim that Ancient Egyptians didn't understand Brain Function?

Can you explain to me HOW "KEMETIC SCHOLARS" make the claim that Ancient Egyptians did have the knowledge or tools to perform anatomy research?

This is the Fall of Dr. Clark & Leonard Jeffries! They have officially fallen, their legacies forever tarnished by choosing Reginald Mabry, to be the Heir to the Intellectual Property.

You got some Nerve!!!

God (the Sun) speaks (emits radio waves) that you hear (absorb and convert) through your antenna (**the spine**). The nerves help distribute this information to the Plasma based Crystal disc, fitted with integrated circuits as well as gates and channels.

How can the eye of Heru and the Djed Pillar be so well known and yet I get attacked for discovering that the Was Scepter is the Aorta?

Light moves around the earth 7 times per second, therefore the number 7 represents the speed of light. The Baboon represents the wisdom of Thoth. We are not the first associate or simply recognize that the Vault of Heaven is Neurochemistry. We are though the first to recognize the Naga as the spiral of the 3rd ventricle, with the "hissing" representing the sound produced by the 3rd ventricle as well as the speed of Light being the

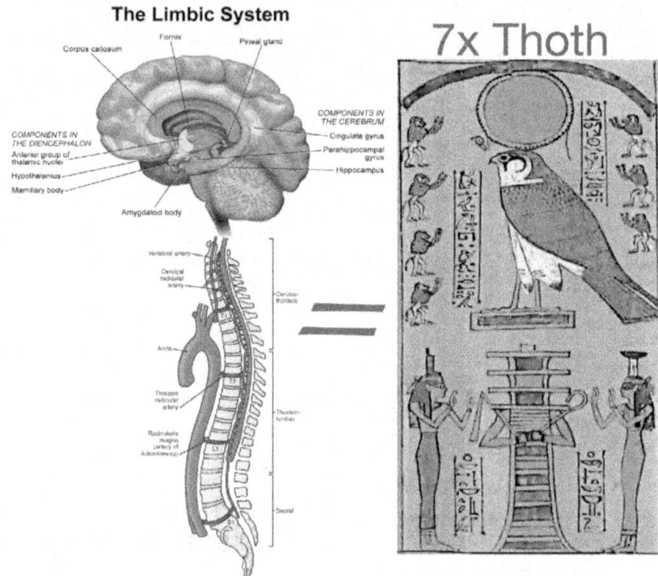

speed of Thoth.

This is how one generation is supposed to build on the last generation's work. We also see the Crook and Flail as the tools God (the Sun) uses to run his flock. His flock being the Red Blood Cells.

The　　　　　　Sun　　　　　　and　　　　　　Earth　　　　　　spe

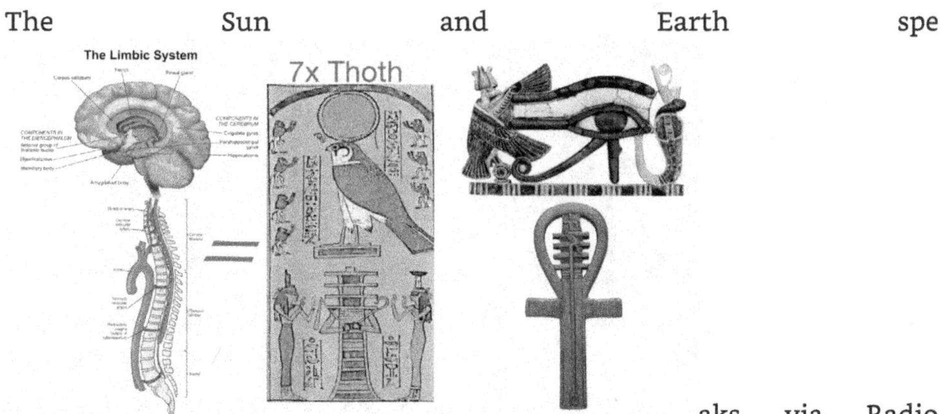

aks via Radio Waves, the radio waves are translated via Schuman Resonances. The Radio Waves are picked up via the Spine, the Spine is the electrical Motherboard as well as a source of Blood Cells.

You got some Nerve!!!

God (the Sun) speaks (emits radio waves) that you hear (absorb and convert) through your antenna (**the spine**). The nerves help distribute this information to the Plasma based Crystal disc, fitted with integrated circuits as well as gates and channels.

How can the eye of Heru and the Djed Pillar be so well known and yet I get attacked for discovering that the Was Scepter is the Aorta?

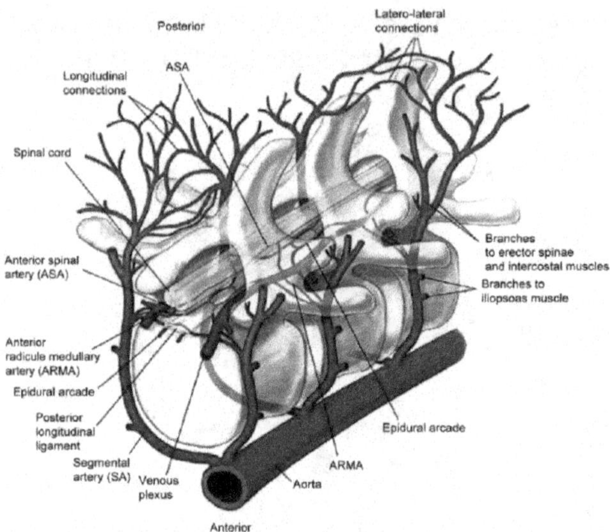

That's the Aorta & Spine from a different angle.

Think about this, the average cell has about 1,000 to 2,500 mitochondria in them versus, the average Nerve/Neuron can have 2,000,000 mitochondria. This is why it is very important to memorize your Time Table from the AlgaRhythm & L'Goat books! The foundation is solid to build on. The very same EnQi cycle feeding electrons to NAD and protons to the F0 motors power Glucose Metabolism & ATP synthesis! Neurons are just more powerful so they require **More Light**.

You got some Nerve!!!

The brain uses over 20% of the body'd total oxygen from the blood! The brain is only 2% of the body's weight, that is a massive amount of energy consumption. 1/4th of that energy is used for background task and 3/4th the energy is used for information processing and neural transmission/ reception.

On average .3 kilowatt hours (kWh) per day per adult, 100x more than what a smartphone uses a day. This translates to 260 calories or 1,088 kilojoules (kJ) a day. The average person's total energy intake is around 8,700 kJ or 2100 kilocalories a day. Now we are full circle back around to the Carb Max Number from the AlgaRhythm book as well as the protein deficit from the Protein Sheik book. Your requires based on your activity and your cholesterol and fat (DHA)... You need cholesterol for building hormones, membranes, Vitamin D etc... You need DHA to build a child's brain, actually DHA and Iodine build new born brains! They are also required to maintain adult brains by creating Neurogenesis, quieting inflammation, protecting Glial cells etc...

Add a new 60 to your Divine Mathematics, the brain is 60% fat! You need fat to maintain your wiring. Fat is the insulation on all your wiring. DHA & **Iodine** help increase Grey Matter in the brain (information processing ability)!

EFAs are more though then just Omega 3 or DHA... You have two types of **Omega 3, Omega 6, Omega 7, Omega 9** etc... There are many types of healthy fats!

GABA quiets and relaxes the Brain. GABA metabolizes sugar look Insulin, GABA functions with Amylin but take note, DHA and GABA should not be taken at the same time. GABA & DHA neutralize one another. They both Relax and Soothe Nerves/Neurons but be mindful to use them separately.

You got some Nerve!!!

God (the Sun) speaks (emits radio waves) that you hear (absorb and convert) through your antenna (**the spine**). The nerves help distribute this information to the Plasma based Crystal disc, fitted with integrated circuits as well as gates and channels.

How can the eye of Heru and the Djed Pillar be so well known and yet I get attacked for discovering that the Was Scepter is the Aorta? How did they eye of Heru wind up an exact replica of the 4 ventricles if they had no knowledge or tools to examine the Brain?

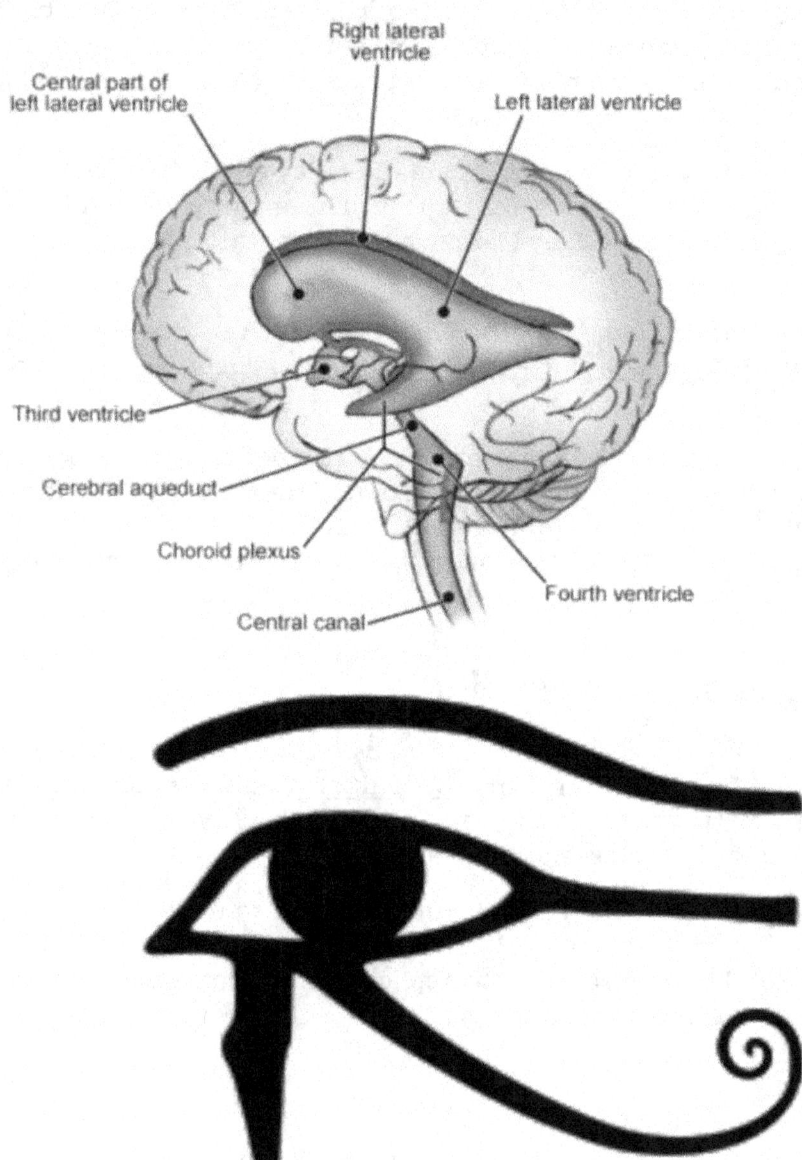
Right lateral
ventricle
Central part of
left lateral ventricle
Left lateral ventricle
Third ventricle
Cerebral aqueduct
Choroid plexus
Fourth ventricle
Central canal

HEARTLY BURNING FAT

We discussed the use of Glycogen and Fat for energy in Melanin vs Diabetes book 4, both are converted to glucose for ATP. Each glucose requires oxygen to be formed, and then at least 4 oxygen atoms to remove the 2 single carbon atoms left behind. The faster your Carbon waster is removed after breaking down glucose the better your endurance etc…

Your nose and lungs offset the work load of the Heart. The better your nose and lungs work, the easier the Heart's job of pumping is. The pulmonary membrane and the iron in the blood help this process as well.

Keep in Polar Haplotypes store their fat first around their organs and secondarily in the skin, Equatorial Haplotypes are the opposite, we store fat around in our Skin First and then the organs. This is how your fat will be burned as well. Polar Haplotypes burn their fat first from around their skin and secondarily in the organs, Equatorial Haplotypes are the opposite, we burn fat first around our organs and then the skin. Get it?

Our Primary Fat Storage site is our Last Reserve to be tapped!

This also means that you need to be mindful of what your body likes. Our Primary Fuel Source is the First to be tapped! Equatorial Haplotypes tap Carbs, Polar Haplotypes tap Fat, primarily. All people burn sugar and fat, we are just outlining preferences and how they play out in real time.

One gram of carbohydrate contains 4 calories (16.7 kilojoules) of energy, 1 gram of fat contains 9 calories (37.6 kilojoules). Glycogen has less and energy but is burned twice as fast. In the past it was taught to strictly focus on your max heart rate because high intensity workouts did not burn fat, they were wrong. HIIT Training depletes sugar storage waaaay faster forcing your body to clear fat sooner!

The old idea of low intensity training for fat burning while true, paints a false narrative about HIIT! The bottom line is that High Intensity Interval Training is more efficient than low intensity training!

These are just add-ons for your programming, this is to help complete what your building from the Gold Book, the Fiscal Edition, Divine Mathematics & the AlgaRhythm books.

Sweating should not be taken as a sign of Fatloss more like Waterloss. Excess waterloss can be dangerous, especially when the electrolytes and nutrients lost during sweating are not re-consumed very quickly.

Sweat is very costly and many make the mistake of 1 believing they can re-hydrate with plain water and 2 thinking sweat = fat burned. This is where you need to mind your vitamins as well! Fat loss means Fat Soluble Vitamins losses and Waterloss means Water Soluble Vitamins are lost.

I just have to ask you, seeing as how these Great Black Scholars and their progeny seem to think Black Biochemistry is unimportant, when Health Issues are the largest cause of death and financial ruin….. How!!!

You got some Nerve!!!

God (the Sun) speaks (emits radio waves) that you hear (absorb and convert) through your antenna (**the spine**). The nerves help distribute this information to the Plasma based Crystal disc, fitted with integrated circuits as well as gates and channels.

How can the eye of Heru and the Djed Pillar be so well known and yet I get attacked for discovering that the Was Scepter is the Aorta?

Heart Disease and Brain Disease are the #1 & #2 killers around the world! The thing they have in common is Nerves/Neurons. To go a step further the Heart and Brain Cells have over 2,000,000 million Mitochondria verses 2,000 in the rest of the body?

Could the problem be the fact that we are all being treated as Primates?

Primates have most of their mitochondria distribution and skeletal muscle are totally different! Primates, and when I say primates, I distinguish us as humans. Primates are design to utilize almost all of their skeletal muscle. I am talking about motor unit recruitment. Humans on the weaker side can recruit 15%-25% of the motor units in skeletal muscle, the strongest humans can recruit 30%-40% of the motor units in muscle tissue.

This highly specific so that we can use what our brains design. We are a more advanced creature. If we see creations as a continuous process and god (or the environment) creating more complex creatures as information gets stored, we can logically have multiple creations of humans and separation of humans from primates. Science supports our theories here.

Human Motor Neurons are parallel to their respective muscle fibers, Primates Motor Neurons cross over their muscle fibers. We aren't designed to full exploit our power without knowledge. A primate is designed in a way that they can be "dumb" strong, humans are not! We are designed for knowledge. We must learned to manage our breath and cardio to maximize our muscle recruitment. We have to learn to manage Myostatin and Follistatin to maximize our muscle recruitment.

A primate can not utilize tools they way we can, they do not have the dexterity or **NERVE CONTROL** for brain or heart surgery!

The spine is special and there is a reason that the ancient used the Snake to Symbolize the Spine. It's Anatomy not magical spells or gobbledegook!

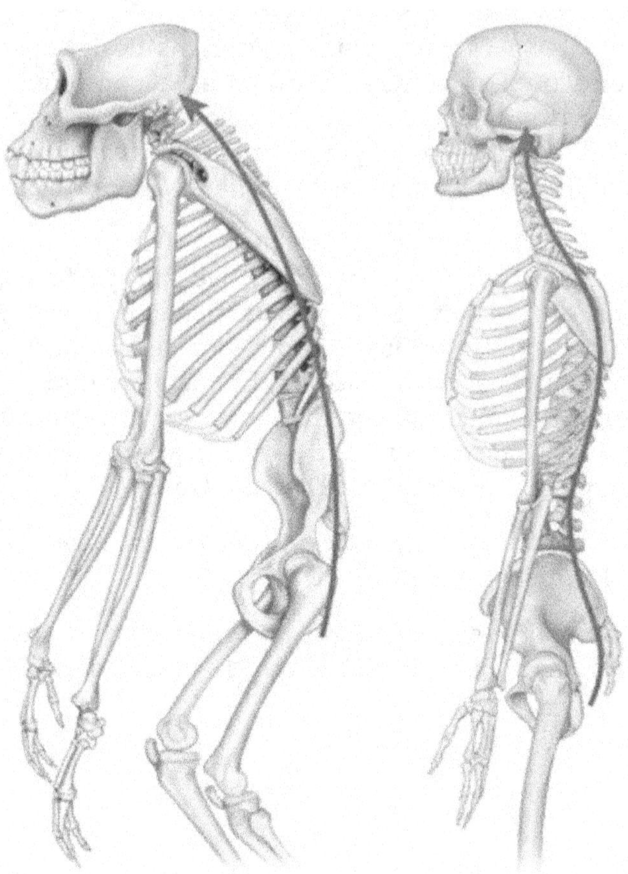

A primates spine makes a wide Arc where as a human spine is Wavy, like the body of a Snake. Why don't these Race Hustling Scholars like Reginald know this or teach information? If he is in fact studying the Djed Pillar?

You see therein lies the twist (pun intended), they believe that studying the Djed Pillar means looking at pictures or Mdu Ntr!!! Noooooooo!!! Once you learn that the Djed Pillar is the Spine, THEN YOU MUST STUDY THE SPINE TO STUDY THE DJED PILLAR, GET IT????

The curve in our spine is designed to support our weight on two feet! Many would say "as infants our spines resemble monkeys"… No! If that's the case you can point to the fish, reptiles etc.. that we resemble as our embryos develop. That means nothing except that the Bible was correct in telling the story of our cellular development.

Primates have mush more fast twitch muscle than we do, we have particular muscles designed for walking on our two feet, these are oxidative because they are in use all day everyday.

Myostatin inhibits muscular healing and growth, to the extent of your daily needs. Follistatin binds up myostatin, promoting muscular growth even without their need or use.

Humans have a heavy expression of myostatin, to keep their muscle development tied directly to muscle usage, this is why humans have much lower muscular density.

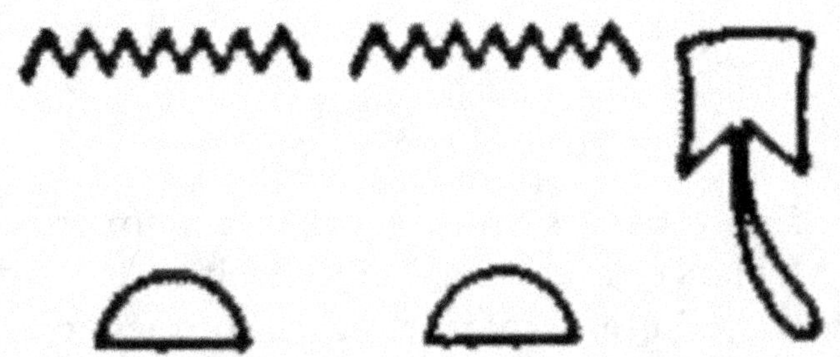

"Membrane" enveloping the Brain

"Coverings of the Brain."

I just want to look at this one again... Could this instead be describing the actual Neurons???

We may need to start a complete Electrician Series after this one???

The Importance of Peripheral Nerves in Adipose Tissue for the Regulation of Energy Balance

Magdalena Blaszkiewicz,[1] Jake W. Willows,[2] Cory P. Johnson,[1] and Kristy L. Townsend[1,2,*]
Author information Article notes Copyright and License information PMC Disclaimer

Abstract

Brown and white adipose tissues are essential for maintenance of proper energy balance and metabolic health. In order to function efficiently, these tissues require both endocrine and neural communication with the brain. Brown adipose tissue (BAT), as well as the inducible brown adipocytes that appear in white adipose tissue (WAT) after simulation, are thermogenic and energy expending. This uncoupling protein 1 (UCP1)-mediated process requires input from sympathetic nerves releasing norepinephrine. In addition to sympathetic noradrenergic signaling, adipose tissue contains sensory nerves that may be important for relaying fuel status to the brain. Chemical and surgical denervation studies of both WAT and BAT have clearly demonstrated the role of peripheral nerves in browning, thermogenesis, lipolysis, and adipogenesis. However, much is still unknown about which subtypes of nerves are present in BAT versus WAT, what nerve products are released from adipose nerves and how they act to mediate metabolic homeostasis, as well as which cell types in adipose are receiving synaptic input. Recent advances in whole-depot imaging and quantification of adipose nerve fibers, as well as other new research findings, have reinvigorated this field of research. This review summarizes the history of research into adipose innervation and brain–adipose communication, and also covers landmark and recent research on this topic to outline what we currently know and do not know about adipose tissue nerve supply and communication with the brain.

Keywords: adipose innervation, BAT, WAT, thermogenesis, sympathetic, brain–adipose communication, adipose peripheral nerves, adipose neuropathy, neural plasticity

1. Introduction

The brain, and chiefly the hypothalamus, is responsible for coordinating energy balance by integrating signals coming from the periphery. These signals include important endocrine hormones and nutrients from the circulatory system, but also feedback from sensory nerves in peripheral tissues and organs. In turn, the brain can communicate outwardly to these tissues and organs through distinct efferent peripheral nerves, such as sympathetic nerves. For adipose tissue, this incoming sympathetic drive and resulting release of the neurotransmitter norepinephrine (NE) is critical for metabolic processes including lipolysis, adipogenesis, and browning. In recent years, several research groups (including ours) have reinvigorated the study of how neural innervation of adipose tissue is regulated, and many new discoveries and advancements in tissue imaging have been made. Lessons from non-adipose tissues, and also from other research animal models, have contributed important knowledge about how peripheral nerves are regulated, including by crosstalk with nearby immune cells that are capable of impacting neural plasticity. Adipose tissue innervation has been studied since the 1890s, and seminal studies were contributed by several research groups in the last few decades. In this review we summarize historic, landmark, and recent studies that provide insights into the roles of adipose tissue nerves in metabolic function.

2. Innervation of Adipose Tissues

2.1. Innervation of Brown Adipose Tissue (BAT)

The notion that neural innervation exists in adipose tissues is not a new one; from an anatomical and functional perspective, all tissues of the body should be innervated—an idea supported since at least the late 1800s. Cardiac tissue and blood vessels were found to be widely innervated, as well as pericardial white adipose tissue (WAT; which is a very "brown" depot), in small rodents as early as the 1890s [1]. Direct evidence of innervation of brown adipose tissue (BAT; in mice and rats) was demonstrated in the mid-20th century [2]. Interestingly, even in the 1950s, Sidman and Fawcett made a statement that would be equally relevant today. They wrote, "Relatively little attention has been paid in recent years to the influence of the nervous system on adipose tissue even though detailed experimental studies on this subject are to be found in the (literature)." They went on to cite a number of studies in the 1930s that presented evidence for the importance of adipose nerves; and themselves stated that mixed nerve types innervate BAT and that many nerve fibers were not associated with blood vessels but extended into the parenchymal space and made direct contact with adipose cells [2]. Similarly timed investigations argued, with the support of fluorescent microscopy, that the sympathetic innervation found in BAT was restricted to the vasculature and was mainly vasoregulatory in function [3]; although, the existence of parenchymal nerve fibers in adipose tissue was at least becoming more accepted a year later [4].

Soon after, Bargmann et al. [5], in the late 1960s, used electron microscopy to demonstrate (in mice, rats, and hedgehogs) that not only did sympathetic fibers envelope BAT vasculature but that they also extended into the parenchymal space. Interestingly, as we describe below, this parenchymal innervation of adipose was rediscovered in recent years with whole-depot imaging techniques. Bargmann et al. [5] were also able to see both non-myelinated and myelinated paravascular (their anatomical term) nerve bundles, but more importantly, they found that small unmyelinated axons were tightly associated with fat cells themselves. Interestingly, the axon terminals of these nerves, some of which were "embedded in invaginations" of the adipocyte surface, contained synaptic vesicles that the authors presumed to contain catecholamines [5]. This presumption was based on the mounting evidence for catecholamine release driving adaptive thermogenesis in BAT in multiple mammalian species [6,7,8], findings which also underscored that NE was essential for this process instead of the previously hypothesized epinephrine/adrenaline [9,10].

Based on these studies, it became accepted that cold-induced thermogenesis caused an increase of NE release to BAT, which resulted in lipolysis and activation of uncoupling protein 1 (UCP1). However, if we look back to some of the original findings regarding adipose innervation [4], there may be another mechanism to consider. Early fluorescent microscopy imaging of BAT and WAT innervation argued for numerous nerve fibers surrounding the vasculature, predominantly around arteries and arterioles [3,4]. Given this perspective, an alternative hypothesis could be that cold-induced thermogenesis does not result in an increase in the concentration of circulating NE, nor might it result in an increase in direct sympathetic drive to WAT and synaptically released NE. Instead there could be stimulation of vasodilation to tissues due to vasoregulatory innervation and thus no resulting change in the absolute catecholamine levels delivered to the tissue per volume of blood, but rather an increased volume of blood that would thereby deliver more catecholamines. This idea could provide a vascular mechanism for how obese adipose tissues loses thermogenic capacity, given the vasculature damage that occurs due to chronic inflammation and the relative loss of vascular supply to adipocytes, due to expanding adipose mass coupled with a lack of new angiogenesis, as reviewed by Stapleton et al.

[11].

These early microscopy studies could not benefit from the use of fluorescently-labeled antibodies targeting markers of sympathetic innervation, as they did not yet exist, thus instead they employed formaldehyde gas to form highly fluorescent isoquinoline derivatives, formed from the presence of monoamines (including NE) [4]. The resulting observations indicated the presence of neurotransmitters in axon terminals of BAT and WAT nerves, and may have actually been a more specific result than what we get with antibody staining today, given the potential for off-target and non-specific binding of the antibodies. The downside of this formaldehyde gas technique was the inability to distinguish the subtype of monoamine they were fluorescing.

2.2. Innervation of White Adipose Tissue (WAT)

The observation of Bargmann et al. [5] that each adipocyte comes in contact with nerve fibers in the parenchyma is consistent with what we and others have recently reported in WAT [12,13,14]. Earlier studies using True Blue as a retrograde neural tracer (crystal implants in WAT) showed sensory innervation in inguinal subcutaneous WAT (i-scWAT), as evidenced by tracing back to the T13/L1-L3 dorsal root ganglia (DRG) [15]. The anterograde transneuronal viral tract tracer, the H129 strain of the herpes simplex virus-1 (HSV-1), has also been used to trace sensory nerve projections from i-scWAT and intraperitoneal epididymal WAT (eWAT), through the same T13/L1 DRG in Siberian hamsters [16]. Together, these studies and others like them have indicated that adipose has bi-directional communication with the brain— through both afferent sensory fibers and efferent sympathetic fibers. However, the role of sensory innervation in WAT continued to be largely understudied in lieu of sympathetic nervous system (SNS) innervation studies in the intervening years. This made sense given the importance of NE for thermogenesis and lipolysis.

More recently, new studies have revisited the function of adipose sensory nerves. Long-form leptin receptor (ObRb) was found on DRG neurons traced from i-scWAT, suggesting leptin could potentially communicate with sensory nerves in adipose via the DRG [17]. Furthermore, SNS-stimulated lipolysis, as well as intra-adipose injection of free fatty acids, such as eicosanoidpentaenoic acid (EPA) and arachidonic acid (AA), could increase adipose afferent nerve activity [18]. This was capable of triggering BAT thermogenesis, an effect that was abolished with surgical denervation of i-scWAT [18].

Although early microscopy studies provided evidence of WAT innervation and hypothesized that these nerves were of SNS origin [4], irrefutable proof of SNS innervation of WAT came from the seminal studies of Youngstrom and Bartness, who demonstrated bidirectional innervation of WAT [19]. Using the retrograde fluorescent tract tracer FluoroGold injected into i-scWAT and eWAT, as well as the anterograde fluorescent tract tracer DiI, they determined that the SNS ganglia also at T13/L1-L3 innervated both fat pads. These studies further showed that there was innervation of the adipocytes themselves, and not just the blood vessels within a depot, as had been previously demonstrated in the mid 1900s. The specificity of the tracing was confirmed by surgical denervation of the fat depots and by injecting the tracers directly into blood vessels. Furthermore, using pseudorabies virus (PRV) retrograde tracing from i-scWAT, which can only trace sympathetic neurons that are synaptically connected, they could create hierarchical connectome that mapped neuronal pathways from the tissue to the brain [20]. For the next two decades, the work of Timothy Bartness would continue to pioneer our understanding of adipose innervation in rodent models [21].

Go to:

3. Lessons from Adipose Denervation Studies

Multiple methods for and consequences of denervation of WAT and BAT have been reported in the literature, and have been described in detail in recent reviews [22,23]. Of these, surgical denervation is considered the most effective at eliminating total neural input and output, as the nerve bundles innervating the tissue are physically resected. However, surgical denervation is generally non-specific to nerve type (as sensory and sympathetic nerve bundles tend to travel together), can be a technically challenging method, and can cause undesirable effects as nerve bundles that innervate adipose depots often innervate other tissues and can run along the vasculature. An alternative approach is chemical denervation. Chemical denervation can provide a selective and localized means of removing nerve supply to WAT depots. The first selective chemical denervation drug was 6-hydroxydopamine (6-OHDA) [24], which is taken up into NE storage vesicles leading to oxidative damage to the membrane and nerve degeneration, and thereby producing a reversible denervation of sympathetic nerves while leaving sensory nerves intact [22]. Later, some chemical denervation studies were undertaken using guanethidine to produce chemical sympathectomy. This drug works by displacing NE from postganglionic sympathetic nerve endings, and decreases reuptake of NE by nerve terminals. When locally administered, it can deplete a tissue of NE, effectively depleting sympathetic tone. It has been used to provide direct evidence of the role of NE in WAT, as local injection of guanethidine to i-scWAT resulted in increased fat pad size, due to adipocyte hyperplasia, in Siberian hamsters [25]. This denervation experiment helped provide a mechanism by which the SNS regulates body mass, which is to regulate adipocyte dynamics and cell size. The current preferred sympathetic denervation drug is 6-OHDA, as subsequent preparations of guanethidine proved less reliable [23].

For chemical denervation of sensory nerves, capsaicin is typically used, which activates vanilliod receptors on unmyelinated and myelinated sensory nerves. The over-activation of the receptors causes an influx of calcium and sodium resulting in an excitotoxic effect [22]. The efficacy of capsaicin-mediated sensory denervation is validated by a reduction in calcitonin gene-related peptide (CGRP) and Substance P content, and although it is not as effective as surgical denervation, this method does appear to leave sympathetic efferent nerves intact [26].

3.1. Denervation of BAT

Some of the most elegant studies demonstrating the importance of neural control for adipose tissue metabolism and function involved surgical denervation of BAT. By removing the neural supply to the organ, observed metabolic perturbations were directly linked to a lack of brain–adipose communication. Indirect evidence for sympathetic control of lipolysis had been demonstrated by studies showing an increased rate of NE turnover (NETO) in both BAT and WAT following cold exposure in rats [27]. Increased NETO in WAT has also been demonstrated with fasting in rats [28]. Denervation studies have added credence to these findings. Unilateral and bilateral denervation of interscapular (iBAT) is technically less difficult than denervation of WAT depots, as nerve bundles innervating iBAT are more easily visualized and anatomically defined (five intercostal nerves that unilaterally innervate iBAT) [29] than those innervating WAT depots [23], and originate mainly from the stellate ganglion [30]. Bilateral denervation of iBAT resulted in greatly impaired thermogenesis and reduced overall energy expenditure, increased body fat mass [31], and "whitening" of the tissue [32]. Furthermore, experiments with unilateral iBAT denervation showed decreased presence of tyrosine hydroxylase (TH) [32] and UCP1 [33] only in the denervated fat pad compared to the intact contralateral pad. In studies where sympathetic drive to BAT increased total energy expenditure, surgical denervation blunted the effect [32,34]. This surgical denervation of BAT was done by severing the large nerve bundles transiting to BAT, as anatomically defined [29], while leaving nearby vasculature intact [35]. Furthermore, bilateral chemical sympathectomy of iBAT increased NETO in i-scWAT [35], demonstrating adipose tissue crosstalk with the brain in the attempt to reestablish energy homeostasis. Chemical denervation of sensory innervation to iBAT also impaired thermogenesis [36], demonstrating the need for sensory feedback from iBAT for proper thermogenic function.

3.2. Denervation of WAT

There are metabolically relevant consequences of losing the nerve supply to WAT. Surgical denervation of WAT led to increased fat pad mass and white adipocyte proliferation and differentiation, as demonstrated in both rats [37] and Siberian hamsters [19,38,39]. The i-scWAT fad pad is innervated by multiple nerve bundles entering the tissue at multiple locations. Surgical denervation of i-scWAT was accomplished by tracking these nerves under four-times magnification to their terminal location and bisecting the nerves at that area [19]. Retroperitoneal WAT (rWAT) is perhaps more easily surgically denervated by lifting the kidney and cutting the three nerve bundles right before they enter the fat pad [38]. These experiments underscored the importance of innervation for regulating hypertrophy versus hyperplasia, as well as for controlling levels of lipolysis. However, surgical denervation could not reveal which nerves are most essential in maintaining proper body mass and metabolic health, as the technique denervates both sympathetic and sensory nerves and causes disturbance of vasculature.

The Bartness lab and others have subsequently used chemical denervation to gain a deeper understanding of which nerves act in adipose depots and how. Chemical symapathectomy (with 6OHDA) of one fat pad increased total body fat and increased adipocyte number in the contralateral fat pad in rats and mice [40]. One interpretation of these data would be that sensory feedback from the denervated pad led to effects in the non-denervated pad via the central nervous system. However, treatment with peripherally-administered leptin could reduce fat pad size independent of innervation status [40], confirming that endocrine and neuronal effects mediate adiposity. In subsequent studies, 6-OHDA denervation of sympathetic nerves in one or both fat depots reduced the NE content and inhibited NETO in other WAT pads as well as in iBAT [41].

Over and over, sympathetic denervation of WAT resulted in increased depot mass, characterized by an increase in cell number and a decrease in lipolysis, as recently reviewed [22]. On the other hand, sensory denervation of iWAT and eWAT increased fat pad mass via hypertrophy instead of hyperplasia, providing a means of differential control of WAT by sympathetic versus sensory nerves [26,39]. The next step in our understanding must be to delineate how different neuropeptides and neurotransmitters exert these effects, and whether sensory nerve products potentially modulate the effects of NE from SNS nerves.

3.3. Potential for Nerve-Independent Thermogenesis in Brown Adipocytes

While the contribution of adipose innervation is clearly important for the regulation of metabolism and thermogenesis, and mice lacking beta-adrenergic receptors cannot easily survive the cold, several studies have attempted to clarify cell-autonomous effects that may circumvent neural inputs to regulate these processes. As is nicely reviewed in [42], beta-adrenergic signaling has differential effects on lipolysis, including activity of the enzymes hormone sensitive lipase (HSL) and adipose triglyceride lipase (ATGL). Non-adrenergic biomolecules can also impact lipolysis through actions on G-protein coupled receptors that act through similar intracellular pathways as adrenergic signaling (e.g., adenylyl cyclase, cAMP). Numerous of these have known neural functions as well, such as purine nucleosides (adenosine), melanocortins, glucocorticoids, and parathyroid hormone. Other receptor-independent pathways to lipolysis have also been uncovered, as well as alternate sources to produce intracellular free fatty acids as a means to activate UCP1 (also reviewed in [42]). What is less convincing; however, is the ability of brown adipocytes to directly sense cold temperature themselves. Cold stimulation has been well-described as stimulating TRP channels on skin sensory nerves, which send signals back to the brain, which leads to coordinated regulation of sympathetic outflow to stimulate thermogenesis. Cold-sensing mechanisms have not been described in a cell autonomous manner, although at least one study has reported a cold-stimulated in vitro culture condition was sufficient to turn on brown adipocyte genes, including UCP1, in cultured 3T3-F442A cells [43]. The underlying reason for this observation may have been cold stress instead of cold-induced thermogenesis, but the mechanism was not fully explored. Mice lacking the beta-adrenergic receptors were still able to stimulate a thermogenic program in scWAT, although the contribution of non-adrenergic nerve products was not explored as a potential mechanism [43].

4. Advancements in Imaging/Analysis Techniques for Visualizing Adipose Innervation

4.1. What Has Been Learned from Tissue Sectioning

To visualize and better understand the anatomy and physiology of adipose tissue, researchers have been processing adipose tissues in micron-thick sections for subsequent histological staining on slides or floating sections [3]. By this method, it is beneficial to stain for multilocularity, browning and UCP1 expression, or the presence of macrophages in crown-like structures. However, adipose innervation is not easily demonstrated in 7–10 μM thick sections because cross-sections of nerves appear mostly as puncta. This does not allow for the quantification of the total tissue innervation and also does not allow for adequate visualization of synapses. This is especially true as we now know that the innervation of WAT is heterogeneous in nature [12,13,14]. Given the significant interest in the innervation of adipose tissue that has recently re-emerged, it is; therefore, important to develop whole-tissue methods for visualizing and quantifying adipose innervation across a depot. The sympathetic innervation of BAT tissue has been well established due to its role in thermogenesis [44,45,46,47]. Conversely, WAT has been relatively understudied as a tissue of significant innervation, and these tools could help increase our knowledge.

Several investigations have been conducted in the past 20 years that have used histological processing of thin-sectioned adipose tissue to elucidate the various nerve types residing there. Immunofluorescence imaging of thin tissue sections using TH as a marker for sympathetic nerve activity has been used extensively to document sympathetic innervation within both WAT [39,48,49,50] and BAT [51]. Tyrosine hydroxylase is the rate-limiting step in catecholamine synthesis and its expression goes up upon sympathetic nerve activation. Immunohistochemical staining for TH in subcutaneous and visceral adipose depots has been used to show an increase in tyrosine hydroxylase immunoreactive (TH+) SNS parenchymal nerve fibers after cold stimulation [51,52]. However, TH immunoreactivity is not a good method for assessing total innervation, as the levels of this enzyme fluctuate in response to SNS stimulation.

It is well known that cold exposure can induce sympathetic drive in both WAT and BAT [53], accompanied by increased TH levels [54] and increased browning and UCP1 expression in WAT [55]. Interestingly, this drive was shown to be greater in females due to an increased expression of estrogen-dependent sympathetic nerves [56]. Warm temperatures elicit the opposite effect in BAT, thus decreasing sympathetic nerve activity and TH expression [57].

Sensory innervation has also been well established in adipose by marking afferent sensory nerves with their neuropeptide products, such as CGRP [39,50,58] and Substance P [50,58]. Both of these neuropeptides are associated with inflammation brought on by sensory nerve nociception [59,60], but it is still unclear what stimulates their secretion in WAT or BAT and how these might affect energy balance.

Studies conducted on rat BAT [61] have shown that only a small subset of brown adipose depots are parasympathetically innervated: pericardial BAT and mediastinal BAT [62]. There is; however, some uncertainty surrounding whether or not WAT is parasympathetically innervated. A study conducted in 2004 suggested the presence of parasympathetic nerves by using retrograde trans-neuronal tracer PRV to mark parasympathetic nerves in rats [63]. This was later refuted when WAT sections failed to be labeled by parasympathetic postganglionic nerve markers, including vesicular acetylcholine transporter (VAChT), vasoactive intestinal protein (VIP), and neuronal nitric oxide synthase (nNOS) in Siberian hamsters [64]. It was proposed by Berthoud et al. [65] that the significant vagal innervation findings were due to leaking of the retrograde tracer and improper controls, thus creating false positives. Kreier and Buijs [66] stated, in a letter to the editor, that the lack of VAChT, VIP, and nNOS staining is inadequate to rule out the significance of parasympathetic input in the WAT due to their highly variable nature within tissues known to have significant parasympathetic input, suggesting that there are no known universally-expressed parasympathetic markers that are equally expressed among all tissue types. They also questioned the ability of Giordano et al. [64] to perform a completely thorough chemical sympathectomy in WAT, stating that mechanical sympathectomy is required. This was soon followed by a rebuttal by Berthoud et al. [67] which argued against the possibility of a parasympathetically innervated tissue showing complete absence of all the markers in question. Giordano et al. [68] also rebutted Kreier and Buijis's statements in a response aptly titled: *Reply to Kreier and Buijs: no sympathy for the claim of parasympathetic innervation of white adipose tissue.* In the decade since, little data have served to clear up the confusion.

4.2. Whole-Tissue Processing and Imaging

The need for whole-tissue (or, whole-mount) imaging techniques became necessary as researchers wished to further their knowledge of neuronal interactions and the extent of synaptic connections within adipose tissues. Given the high lipid content in adipose and the brain, the autofluorescence of lipids was problematic in imaging these particular tissues in toto. Accordingly, a technique was needed to remove lipids from the tissue or blunt lipid autofluorescence. To chemically delipidate the tissue, methods were pursued to optically clear the tissues in order to reduce tissue autofluorescence and limit light adsorption, while having minimal effects on tissue morphology [69].

Since as early as 1911, clearing techniques have been implemented in various histological studies. Widely accepted to be the first clearing method published was a benzyl alcohol-methyl salicylate mixture used to aid in the visualization of anastomoses between coronary arteries in the heart [70]. Disappointingly, this method caused significant tissue deformity and damage due to excessive tissue shrinkage and superficial necrosis [71]. This clearing technique also lacked the crucial delipidation step that would be necessary for lipid-rich tissues such as the brain or adipose.

The first clearing method that included delipidation was a method originally developed for whole brains using benzyl alcohol/benzyl benzoate (BABB) [72]. This technique was slightly modified and used in the first published whole-tissue imaging study of adipose innervation conducted on mouse i-scWAT [12].

Several groups concurrently worked to develop similar protocols for adipose tissue whole-mount imaging [13,14].

Several other clearing techniques with delipidation have been applied to whole-adipose depots since then, in order to explore innervation. One such technique is iDISCO [73], which is another solvent-based clearing technique that has the added benefit of reducing the antibody fluorescence quenching that was problematic in traditional BABB clearing [74]. iDISCO is the basis for nearly all of the whole-depot clearing techniques currently published for adipose [14,75,76,77,78,79]. This being so, iDISCO, is far from an ideal clearing method. iDISCO has a fluorescent protein emission lifespan longer than that of many other clearing methods but it is still only a couple days long requiring immediate imaging of tissues [69,74]. iDISCO also does not preserve accurate tissue morphology due to tissue shrinkage and tissue hardening [74]. These factors should be a considered for any study that uses iDISCO as a clearing agent.

The iDISCO clearing technique was further modified for use in adipose by the addition of a more thorough methanol/ dichloromethane-based delipidation step. This adipose specific method has been termed Adipo-Clear [14,79]. Clearing techniques are continuing to evolve and have moved from clearing entire organs to clearing entire organisms [80,81] and will continue to be implemented in adipose-nerve studies as time moves on. Similar whole-tissue imaging techniques have even been applied to engineered adipose substitutes to allow for characterization of the vascular networks that reside in them [82].

The aforementioned clearing techniques as well as many others have been comprehensively reviewed for general tissue use [69,71,74] and for specific use in scWAT [13]. With the noted advancements in clearing techniques and whole-tissue 3D imaging of adipose tissue, it is important to note that clearing is not always necessary. Sudan Black B (which we now call Typogen Black) can be used to block a significant amount of lipid and lipofuscin autofluorescence. TrueBlack® Lipofuscin Autofluorescence Quencher should be used in place of Typogen Black when imaging in a far-red channel, due to its inherent fluorescence at longer wavelengths. Lipid/lipofuscin blocking should be followed by washes with 1X PBS with 10U/mL heparin. Heparin reduces the majority of autofluorescence from the vasculature. Tissue thickness in the z-direction can also be significantly reduced with only slight deformity to the tissue. This can be done by placing the tissue between two glass slides held together by large binder clips for 1.5 h at 4°C [13]. Many of the solvents used for tissue clearing, such as BABB or iDISCO, can be caustic to microscope lenses and the squishing technique stated above can avoid the need for purchasing special BABB safe lenses.

Since the interactions between nerves and vasculature are clearly important, techniques for visualizing adipose vascular supply have been developed, including the use of Isolectin-IB4 [77,83], which binds to group B erythrocytes, perivascular cells, and endothelial cells [84]. Isolectin-IB4 staining has the caveat of staining certain sensory nerves as well as vasculature [85], but stained nerves can be easily distinguished from stained vasculature due to morphology. Isolectin-IB4 staining in whole-mount adipose tissues has been used to show a decrease in adipose depot vascular supply in obese mice [77], and to investigate age-related neuropathy of the nerves surrounding vasculature in i-scWAT [13].

4.3. Discoveries Using Whole-Adipose Tissue Imaging

Many important discoveries have been made to increase our understanding of adipose nerve interactions that would have been impossible without the utilization of whole-tissue imaging techniques. The first study to publish observations on whole-mount adipose innervation did so by embedding a mouse i-scWAT depot in agarose, clearing it in BABB, and imaging the tissue with optical projection tomography before 3D reconstruction. This was the first time whole-depot images were taken that clearly showed vasculature and axon bundles in adipose, which were branching across the length of the tissue. In that same study they also showed adipose–nerve connections within an i-scWAT depot in vivo [12].

Two years later a study was published on i-scWAT innervation that used what the authors called a pan-neuronal marker; synaptophysin, the sympathetic marker TH, and the adipocyte marker perilipin [75]. Although often used as a pan-neuronal marker, synaptophysin is more accurately described as a pre-synaptic marker present on nearly all pre-synaptic vesicles and is limited by not being an actual axonal membrane protein [86,87].

The tissues from mice were optically cleared with a slightly modified iDISCO technique, imaged on a lightsheet microscope, and 3D reconstructed in a process they termed "volume fluorescence imaging." Their findings showed that sympathetic nerve fibers were located in close contact with approximately 91.3% of all adipocytes, something that was first proposed in 1968 [5]. Synaptophysin and TH were 98.8% co-localized [75], which the authors suggested was evidence for the majority of i-scWAT nerves being sympathetic, leaving only 1.2% as a possible sensory and/or parasympathetic type. However, it is unclear whether this co-localization of synpatophysin and TH was observed under basal- or cold-stimulated conditions. Cold stimulation reversibly increases TH+ fiber density in i-scWAT [78] and would likely increase the number of presynaptic vesicles marked by synaptophysin. If these results are from cold stimulated animals then the data are possibly skewed and may be overestimating the ratio of sympathetic to sensory nerves in i-scWAT under basal conditions. This estimate also does not seem to fit with recently published images of sensory innervation of

WAT [13], which demonstrate widespread sensory nerves (marked by Nav1.8) in i-scWAT. Additionally, immunofluorescence labeling of parasympathetic nerve marker ChAT revealed no more than 5 ChAT expressing nerves per i-scWAT depot [75], supporting earlier studies which found little to no parasympathetic fibers in WAT [64].

Further investigation into sympathetic innervation of WAT was conducted using the Adipo-Clear technique and lightsheet microscopy. Mice were cold exposed to elicit sympathetic activity and tissue browning. This study found significant intra-adipose variation in TH+ fibers between subcutaneous and visceral depots [14]. Tissue autofluorescence was used to show tissue morphology in this study [14]. 3D projections of sympathetic (TH +) nerves within both the i-scWAT and eWAT were reconstructed to show differences in arborization between tissue types. Chi et al. [14] described the sympathetic innervation of i-scWAT to be arborized into "discreet lobules", whereas eWAT had an "amorphous structure". It has since been revealed that the inguinal subcutaneous depot has a specific pattern of innervation. The largest nerve bundles, which we are now calling the subiliac transverse nerves, are located at the tissue center, which span the length of the tissue traversing across the subiliac lymphnode in conjunction with the thoracoepigastric vein. It is from these larger nerve bundles that the majority of the smaller nerves branch off from [13].

A number of similar studies have been conducted to investigate whole-adipose innervation with cold challenge. Whole-depot i-scWAT imaging and quantification of the pan-neuronal marker β3-Tubulin [13] and of TH+ nerve fibers in 0.3 mm3 representative sections [78] all suggest an increase in nerve arborization with cold challenge. It has also been shown that i-scWAT innervation returns to the room temperature state following rewarming, as indicated by a drastic reduction of neuronal arbors [13,78].

It is important to note that some of the studies using whole-mount tissue imaging of adipose [75,77,78] only quantify representative 3D-projection images of 0.3 mm3 sections for much of their findings, in lieu of the entire cleared depot. Due to the regional specific arborization patterns in i-scWAT, as previously described [13,14], it is apparent why whole-depot imaging and quantification of innervation is necessary and why representative sections cannot yield completely accurate results.

5. Peripheral Nerve Regulation in the Pancreas, Liver, and Gut

Beyond adipose tissue, numerous peripheral metabolic organs have been used to demonstrate the importance of neural innervation and brain–adipose communication for the regulation of energy balance. Below we summarize recent findings from the pancreas, liver, and gut. Findings from these organs may inform the future study of adipose innervation and brain–adipose communication, as there may be similar mechanisms for regulation of peripheral innervation of these tissues.

5.1. Pancreas

The pancreas contains three primary secretory cell types, α-, β-, and δ-cells, that reside in the Islets of Langerhans and are responsible for the release of metabolic hormones such as glucagon, insulin, and somatostatin, respectively. Pancreatic islets are known to be highly innervated by the peripheral nervous system, particularly from fibers of vagal and celiac ganglion origin [88,89,90]. A discovery outlined in Paul Langerhans' doctoral dissertation in 1869 [89,90] depicted a close relationship between hormone release and peripheral nerves, in this case non-myelinated nerves in rabbit and cat pancreas, with innervation observed in both the islets and the blood vessels proximal to the islets [89,90]. In recent research, humans have been shown to contain sparser innervation of the islets when compared to mice

[91,92,93].

Neural regulation of secretory cells in the pancreas is supported by a number of studies. Acetylcholine, a neurotransmitter released by both sympathetic and parasympathetic nerves, is capable of stimulating hormone secretion in both β-cells and δ-cells [94,95,96]. α-cells are not known to be stimulated by acetylcholine [97] but do express the GABAA receptor, which indicates that these cells may be regulated through inhibitory GABAergic signaling [98,99,100]. Interestingly, Ikegami et al. [101] have also uncovered increased GABAergic signaling in BAT of mice suffering from diet-induced obesity [101].

Diabetic polyneuropathy is a condition characterized by high levels of extracellular glucose, inflammation, and degradation/ death of peripheral nerves, ultimately resulting in tissue necrosis due to lack of proper neural innervation and vascular supply. Neuropathic mechanisms are well documented in dermal layers but are also present in sub-dermal tissues including the pancreas [102], muscle [13,103,104,105], and scWAT [13]. The exact mechanisms mediating pancreatic neuropathy, or the reversal thereof, are not completely understood. However, current research in neuroimmune interactions aims to fill these gaps.

Many studies have shown bi-directional communication between immune cells and peripheral nerves, indicating that neuroimmune interactions play a vital role in the progression of pancreatic diseases. Mast cells, known for their importance in allergy response, are also known to be involved in wound healing. In the pancreas, mast cells are speculated to contribute to neuroplasticity and pain severity by secreting nerve growth factor (NGF), which binds to TrkA receptors on sensory neurons and promotes the expression of Substance P [106,107]. This process is then exacerbated by NGF and Substance P-mediated mast cell recruitment and degranulation, respectively [107]. NGF is also known to be released by many other cell types including other immune cells [108], likely contributing to symptom severity. Demir et al. [109] have presented evidence of mast cells congregating perineurally in the rat pancreas, and Zhu et al. [110] have shown that anti-NGF treatment in a rat model of pancreatitis correlates with decreased nociception.

Interestingly, neurturin, a glial-derived neurotrophic factor, is increased in the human pancreas in chronic pancreatitis (CP), and is characterized by increased neural sprouting. DRG from rat were cultured in medium supplemented with human tissue extracts, prepared from patients with CP, and exhibited increased neurite outgrowth in cultured rat DRG cells when compared to controls [111]. This indicated a correlation between neural sprouting and neurturin levels in the pancreas. In addition, CGRP, Substance P, and Neuropeptide Y are known neuropeptides in the rat pancreas [112]. These peptides are major mediators of neuroimmune interactions in the periphery and are essential to the bidirectional communication seen between nerves and immune cells [108].

5.2. Liver

Hepatic innervation is similar to that of pancreatic innervation. In 1886 Walter Holbrook Gaskell reported, "An enormous number of non-medullated fibers stream out from these large ganglia to the intestines, stomach, liver, kidney..." [113]. These findings were further investigated by his scientific progeny F.H. Edgeworth, using the dog as a model animal; from which he determined that the nerve supply to the liver came primarily from the gastric plexus of the vagus, as well as sympathetic fibers from the celiac ganglia [114]. In 2006, Kreier et al. [115] investigated the interconnectivity of the nerves innervating the liver, pancreas, and adipose. Interestingly, rWAT was found to contain innervation of the same origin as the liver and pancreas, unlike i-scWAT, indicating differential innervation patterns for the two adipose depots and possibly preferential targeting of rWAT, which is known for easily browning, as a primary source of fuel [51].

Neural regulation of liver functions, such as glycogenolysis, the breakdown of glycogen secreted by α-cells in the pancreas into glucose, is variable among mammals. In guinea pigs and humans, sympathetic nerve fibers have been reported to extend intralobularly, ending deep in the parenchyma, while this was found to not be the case in liver of rats and mice [116,117,118]. It was suggested that a plethora of gap junctions among hepatocytes in these models may compensate for the lack of direct sympathetic stimulation [119,120,121]. Considering the speculative nature of these observations, more research is needed to uncover a definitive mechanism for how hepatic innervation affects hepatocyte and liver function.

Regarding neural regulation of liver function, hepatic lipid metabolism was augmented with increased sympathetic drive. One study used a high-fat diet (HFD) supplemented with purified green tea catechins to stimulate sympathetic nerve activity, which led to decreased body weight and increased β-oxidation markers in the liver when compared to normal HFD mice [122]. Hepatic vagal innervation allows for bidirectional communication between the liver and brain, which is accomplished primarily through sensory and parasympathetic nerves. Localized disruption of vagal nerves innervating the liver with kilohertz frequency alternating current (KHFAC) [123,124] has exhibited beneficial metabolic effects in a clinical setting, including improved glycemic control in the human liver [125]. Interestingly, another study found that chemical denervation in the liver using 6-OHDA in rats resulted in impaired liver regeneration after injury but had no effect on liver function [126].

NGF is produced by a variety of cell types including immune cells, such as mast cells and macrophages [108]. In the liver, NGF is one of many signaling molecules used to promote a pro-inflammatory response when secreted by hepatic stellate cells (HSCs) [127]. The secretion of NGF via HSCs is interesting, since they comprise nearly 10% of the liver and are known to function primarily in the formation of scar tissue in response to hepatic injury. Kupffer cells are specialized resident macrophages of the liver that function as phagocytes to remove noxious substances delivered to the liver via the blood. These cells have been shown to express glial fibrillary acidic protein (GFAP), which is known as a mature astroglial marker in the central nervous system, as well as a glial-like marker in the periphery [128]. This again emphasizes the close relationship between glial cells in the brain and immune cells in the periphery. NGF is known to promote neuroplasticity in brain development [129] and in adult peripheral tissues [130]. Therefore, it is not unreasonable to believe that neurotrophic factor signaling plays a role in neural health throughout the liver, or in other peripheral tissues; however, more research must be done to elucidate specific mechanisms implicating NGF actions.

5.3. Gut

As may be expected from the proximity of the pancreas, liver, and gut, the origin of nerves innervating the gut is consistent with those innervating the pancreas and liver. Again, Gaskell in 1886 was a major contributor to the understanding of nerves innervating peripheral tissues, which included the gut [113,114]. One pivotal study that laid the groundwork for further research in this area was published by Hans-Rudolf Berthoud in 1991 [131]. In Berthoud's study, dextran biotin, a bi-directional neuronal tracer, was used to trace nerves innervating the gut, resulting in a comprehensive map of vagal nerves. It was concluded that vagal innervation of the gut is primarily originated from the gastric branch, celiac branch, and a small contribution from the hepatic branch innervating the distal stomach [131].

Current research is investigating nerve sub-types and their roles in proper gut function. Cholecystokinin receptor (CCKR), a known afferent nerve receptor in the gut [132,133], was found to increase expression in the nodose ganglia (NG) of the vagus in response to obesity in high-fat diet fed diet-induced obesity prone (DIO-P) rats [134]. Recently, a method of selective ablation of afferent nerves (deafferentation) was developed, using a ribosomal inactivating protein, saporin (SAP), and CCK together as a conjugate. The SAP–CCK conjugate was unilaterally injected into the NG effectively blocking afferent nerve communication to the brain in rats, which was validated using immunostaining as well as behavioral assays [135]. This method is a useful tool for afferent denervation while sparing efferent fibers. Complementary to SAP–CCK ablation of vagal afferents, de Lartigue et al. [136] selectively deleted leptin receptors on NaV1.8 vagal afferent neurons. Genetic knockout of leptin receptors on sensory nerves in vagal afferents led to increased weight-gain, compared to wild-type controls, by preventing appropriate gut–brain signaling [136]. These studies provide essential evidence for the importance of gut–brain communication through vagal afferent innervation of the gut and their relationship to adipose tissue accumulation; while also complementing previous findings in adipose regarding the presence of the ObRb leptin receptor on DRG nerves innervating i-scWAT [17].

Bi-directional communication between gut resident nerves and immune cells has been an active area of study, and an interesting role for neurotrophic factors has been implicated in the progression and severity of inflammatory responses in the gut. NGF is secreted by a variety of immune cell types in the body including mast cells and macrophages, and promotes a plethora of signaling pathways including anti-inflammatory [108] and survival [108,137]. NGF signaling has also been linked to the expression of known sensory neuropeptides, CGRP and Substance P, in the rat gut [138]; however, the direct source of NGF secretion is not known due to the diversity of cell types capable of its production [108]. Interestingly, NGF also promotes the formation of colonic afferent central terminals (CACTs), which are localized to the dorsal horn of the spinal cord and increase visceral nociception in colitic mice [139].

5.4. Perspective

It is important to note that current research models using rodents to study the pancreas and liver indicate significant differences in the distribution of nerves and nerve types compared to that of humans [91,92,93,116,117,118], which may be problematic in the translation of this research to a clinical setting. Important distinctions have been outlined above regarding these innervation patterns. Although these models are limited in their translational power for human studies, the similarities in functional output of the organ or tissue could still be considered useful for further research of nerve–endocrine–immune interactions, as this cross-talk between physiological systems likely remains conserved. Interestingly, species differences were not as pronounced in models of gut innervation. Moreover, it is known that innervation patterns of the gut are conserved throughout a variety of species that span the breadth of the animal kingdom [140].

6. Adipose Neuroimmune Interactions

Although the role of immune cells, especially macrophages, in adipose tissue has been and continues to be an active area of study, neuroimmune interactions in adipose tissue remain largely obscure. It had been suggested that BAT and WAT macrophages synthesize catecholamines in response to cold [141]. Although Nguyen et al. argued that cold-induced adaptive thermogenesis requires alternatively activated (M2, anti-inflammatory) macrophages and did demonstrate that preventing this macrophage polarization resulted in an impaired thermogenic response, these findings were later challenged to suggest a different explanation for the observed relationship between macrophages and catecholamines. In 2017, Fischer et al. used a mouse model with genetic deletion of TH (the rate limiting enzyme in catecholamine production) in hematopoietic cells [142]. By this method, they refuted the findings that alternatively activated macrophages "synthesize" catecholamines. In their study, not only did deletion of TH in hematopoietic cells have no effect on energy expenditure, RNA sequencing on macrophages from various adipose tissues revealed that none of the macrophage populations tested contained transcripts for TH.

The debate between these two sets of findings may have found its resolution with some recent publications. Studies using zebrafish have demonstrated a role for macrophage signaling over long distances between non-immune cells during tissue developmental remodeling, whereby macrophages transported airineme vesicles between two different cell types [143]. Furthermore, buried in literature from the 1970s, was evidence that mouse peritoneal macrophages accumulated NE in vitro [144]. These studies allow for the possibility of macrophages transporting other materials, such as NE, within adipose tissues.

Soon after, Pirzgalska et al. presented data that supported similar macrophage behavior but pertinent to neuroimmune interactions in adipose tissue [145]. They recently described a distinct macrophage population that associates in a specific manner with SNS nerves of i-scWAT. The appropriately named sympathetic neuron-associated macrophages (SAMs), can be found interacting with SNS fibers within WAT and are not only morphologically distinct from adipose tissue resident macrophages (ATMs), but exhibit a gene expression pattern distinct from adipose and other tissue macrophages [145], including expression of genes related to synaptic signaling, cell–cell adhesion, and neuron development. Unlike the circular morphology of ATMs, SAMs wrap around SNS fibers and exhibit an extended shape with long dendritic like projections. Like observations made by Nguyen et al., SAMs contained significant amounts of intracellular NE, but lacked the requisite enzymes for NE synthesis, as previously reported for macrophages [141,142]. These macrophages were of the Cx3cr1+ lineage and exhibited a pro-inflammatory state more similar to classically-activated than M2-type macrophages; however, their most distinguishing feature was the expression of solute carrier family 6 member 2 (Slc6a2; a known NE transporter), as well as monoamine oxidase A (MAOA), an enzyme that degrades NE. Although other macrophages have been shown to express MAOA [145], only SNS fiber-associating SAMs expressed Slc6a2 [145]. The authors proposed, quite believably, that SAMs were acting as an NE sink, taking up excess NE after SNS stimulation and degrading it. The transport of NE by SAMs was not explored. They also showed that SAMs are recruited to WAT in obesity (both diet-induced and genetic models) and may be contributing to the adipocyte hypertrophy through over-degradation of NE. They went on to show that ablation of Slc6a2 from SAMs in obese mice lead to an obesity rescue, through reestablishment of NE levels that served to increase lipolysis and energy expending processes, such as browning of WAT. SAMs (with analogous molecular machinery) were also identified in the SNS tissue of humans [145]. SAMs have been shown to associate with other neuronal tissues, such as the SCG and thoracic chains, and are also present in BAT [145]. However, their abundance in BAT is much lower than WAT, and their role in BAT may not be as metabolically relevant as it is in WAT, but this remains to be seen.

In a parallel study, Camell et al. presented findings of ATMs in aged mice that degrade NE and contribute to age-related lipolysis impairment in visceral adipose tissue (VAT) [146]. ATMs from 24-month-old mice showed increased expression of MAOA and other catecholamine degrading enzymes in a NOD-, LRR-, and pyrin domain-containing (NLRP)3 inflammasome dependent manner, compared to young three-month-old mice [146]. Furthermore, Camell et al. independently showed that certain ATMs were closely associated with TH+ nerves in VAT [146]; providing the likelihood that what they called nerve-associated macrophages (NAMs) may be the same cells as SAMs. Although Camell et al. used a LysM-Cre:mTmG reporter mouse model to visualize their ATMs, which is a broader myeloid marker than the Cx3cr1+ model Pirzgalska et al. used, they did not investigate whether NAMs expressed Slc6a2 (SAM marker) even though the morphology of their NAMs is consistent with that of SAMs.

Mutations in another type of Cx3cr1+ macrophage that do not appear to be SAMs have been linked to decreased BAT innervation and subsequent loss of homeostatic energy expenditure [147]. Mice with Mecp2 (methyl-CpG-binding protein 2) deficiency in a subset of BAT-resident Cx3cr1+ macrophages, exhibited lower expression of UCP1, a paucity of BAT tissue, and developed obesity after three to four months of age [147]. Interestingly these findings were BAT-specific and no changes were observed in WAT. Furthermore, tamoxifen inducible *Cx3cr1 cre:Mecp2fl/y* mice were created to restrict Mecp2 deficiency from macrophage precursor cells (including brain microglia), and which also allowed for the mutation to be induced at a stage when tissue macrophages were mature. These animals were shown to respond to acute cold challenge, which appeared to rescue the BAT impairment [147]. Mecp2 is an ubiquitously-expressed nuclear transcription regulator [148] that maintains mature neurons and synaptic connectivity [149]. Mecp2 deficient macrophages showed an up-regulation of PlexinA4, which is known to signal through semaphorins to guide axonal growth [150,151]. Wolf et al.; thus, argued that overexpression of PlexinA4 in Mecp2 deficient macrophages inhibits axonal outgrowth in BAT, thus diminishing its function and ability to maintain homeostatic thermogenesis. They did confirm the presence of Sema6A+ neurons in BAT tissue, which supports their working model, as PlexinA4 reverse-signals through Sema6a to inhibit axonal outgrowth [151]. However, the question remains as to what overcomes this axonal inhibition with cold exposure, since acute cold exposure appeared to rescue the impaired phenotype. Cold exposure increases NE content in adipose tissue. Macrophages along with other immune cells express adrenergic receptors that bind NE [152], and have been shown to produce neurotrophic factors such as NGF [153] and brain derived neurotrophic factor (BDNF) [154] in human peripheral blood and the human brain [154], suggesting another possible mechanism in regulation of axonal plasticity may exist in adipose tissue, whereby immune cells are synaptically wired and release neurotrophic factor to nearby nerves.

In most studies mentioned above, it was clear that Cx3cr1+ immune cells are implicated in the neuro–immune interaction in adipose tissue. These findings suggest that multiple subsets of Cx3cr1+ macrophages work in concert to maintain energy homeostasis though interactions with the neural innervation of adipose depots. There are many more studies necessary to fully understand the diversity of these immune cells, and what neuroimmune role Cx3cr1- macrophages may play in adipose tissue, if any. One issue that may have been addressed by the data described above is that definitions such as "classically activated" or "alternatively activated" (i.e., M1 or M2) macrophages are not sufficient labels when describing the diverse populations of macrophages in adipose tissue. This has been well-understood by immunologists for many years, and the adipose field is now catching up to this idea.

7. Perspective

In summary, we are in the midst of an exciting time for the investigation of adipose tissue innervation and brain–adipose neural communication, given the flurry of recent publications providing new insights into innervation patterns, neuroimmune interactions, and regulation of adipose neuropathy and nerve plasticity in adipose depots (Figure 1). In addition, the new research tools that are being developed to genetically ablate nerves from specific tissues, including perhaps distinct adipose depots, as well as new microscopy methods for whole-depot imaging of nerves, will further provide new knowledge regarding how nerve supply is regulated in peripheral metabolic tissues in order to regulate whole-body energy balance and metabolic health.

Key Developments in the Potential of Curcumin for the Treatment of Peripheral Neuropathies

Martial Caillaud,[1,*] Yu Par Aung Myo,[1] Bryan D. McKiver,[1] Urszula Osinska Warncke,[1] Danielle Thompson,[1] Jared Mann,[1] Egidio Del Fabbro,[2,3] Alexis Desmoulière,[4] Fabrice Billet,[4] and M. Imad Damaj[1,3,*]
Author information Article notes Copyright and License information PMC Disclaimer

Abstract

Peripheral neuropathies (PN) can be triggered after metabolic diseases, traumatic peripheral nerve injury, genetic mutations, toxic substances, and/or inflammation. PN is a major clinical problem, affecting many patients and with few effective therapeutics. Recently, interest in natural dietary compounds, such as polyphenols, in human health has led to a great deal of research, especially in PN. Curcumin is a polyphenol extracted from the root of Curcuma longa. This molecule has long been used in Asian medicine for its anti-inflammatory, antibacterial, and antioxidant properties. However, like numerous polyphenols, curcumin has a very low bioavailability and a very fast metabolism. This review addresses multiple aspects of curcumin in PN, including bioavailability issues, new formulations, observations in animal behavioral tests, electrophysiological, histological, and molecular aspects, and clinical trials published to date. The, review covers in vitro and in vivo studies, with a special focus on the molecular mechanisms of curcumin (anti-inflammatory, antioxidant, anti-endoplasmic reticulum stress (anti-ER-stress), neuroprotection, and glial protection). This review provides for the first time an overview of curcumin in the treatment of PN. Finally, because PN are associated with numerous pathologies (e.g., cancers, diabetes, addiction, inflammatory disease...), this review is likely to interest a large audience.

Keywords: curcumin, peripheral neuropathy, antioxidant, anti-inflammatory, anti-ER-stress, clinical trial

1. Introduction

Peripheral neuropathies (PN) can be inherited or acquired as a result of a pathological process or trauma [1]. Causes of acquired PN can have multiple origins such as autoimmune, toxic, alcoholic, diabetic, cancerous, chemo-induced, and traumatic, including crushing, constriction, stretching, and complete nerve sectioning [2,3,4]. However, the precise ethology of some neuropathies is sometimes not identified. Clinicians refer to these conditions as idiopathic neuropathies. PN may affect a single nerve (mononeuropathy), two or more nerves in different areas (multiple mononeuropathy), or many nerves (polyneuropathy). Carpal tunnel syndrome and facial paralysis are examples of mononeuropathy. Most people with PN have polyneuropathy affecting longer nerve fibers (length-dependent polyneuropathy) [5].

The symptomatology is very diverse depending on the type of nerve fibers affected. In the case of sensory fiber damage, symptoms are dependent on the caliber and size of the nerve fibers. These symptoms are generally progressive numbness, tingling in the feet or hands which may extend to the legs and arms, or even sharp, throbbing, icy or burning pain, stinging sensations and extreme sensitivity to touch. In the case of motor fiber damage, the most common symptoms are a lack of motor coordination and falls, muscle weakness or paralysis. If autonomic nerves are affected, signs and symptoms may include: heat intolerance and alterations in sweating, dermal problems, intestinal, bladder or digestive problems, but also changes in blood pressure, which can lead to dizziness [1,2].

The major clinical problem in PN, in addition to the difficulties in diagnosing and understanding pathological mechanisms, is that they are poorly treated with currently available therapeutics.

Recently, interest in the role of dietary antioxidants, such as polyphenols, in human health has led to a great deal of research on their potential as possible treatment of many inflammatory diseases. Among these polyphenols, curcumin which has long been used in traditional Asian cuisine and medicine, is an attractive molecule. However, curcumin has a very low bioavailability and a very fast metabolism. Thus, very high doses are required to achieve therapeutic effects given the uncertainty that curcumin will reach the target organ.

Curcumin [1,7-bis(4-hydroxy-3-methoxyphenyl)-1,6-heptadiene-3,5-dione], also known as diferuloylmethane, is a polyphenol present in the rhizome of Curcuma longa [6]. Curcuma longa powder is a spice known as turmeric and used in the preparation of curry. Turmeric powder is an orange-yellow crystalline compound that is used as a food coloring agent [6]. Traditionally, turmeric powder has been used in Asian countries as a medicinal preparation to combat several diseases because of its antioxidant [7], anti-inflammatory [6], antimicrobial [8], anticancer [9], and neuroprotective [10] properties. Over the past 50 years, it has been shown that most of the effects of Curcuma longa are primarily due to curcumin, with potential beneficial properties against diabetes, allergies, arthritis, neuropathies, and other chronic diseases [11]. However, there are other components of Curcuma longa that, together with curcumin, form the curcuminoid group [12]. These are demethoxycurcumin and bis-demethoxycurcumin. The curcuminoid group constitutes about 5% of the total components of Curcuma longa and curcumin is the most abundant of this group with 77% [12].

This review provides an update that is focused on pre-clinical and clinical studies investigating the use of curcumin in the treatment of PN and evaluating future therapeutic opportunities.

Go to:

2. Curcumin Solubility, Kinetics, Bioavailability, and Metabolism

2.1. Solubility and Stability

The therapeutic potential of curcumin is restricted by a low solubility in aqueous solution, chemical instability, and unfavorable pharmacokinetic properties (ADME: absorption, distribution, metabolism and excretion). Due to its lipophilic nature, curcumin is practically insoluble in aqueous solution at room temperature and neutral pH [13,14]. Therefore, the use of organic solvents (such as methanol, ethanol, acetone, or dimethyl sulfoxide) is usually required. Moreover, curcumin is relatively unstable. At both neutral and alkaline pH, it degrades quickly into various compounds including ferulic acid, feruloyl methane, vanillin, and autoxidation products (bicyclopentadione primarily) [15,16,17,18]. In addition, curcumin is also sensitive to light in both solid and solubilized forms [19].

2.2. Bioavailability

The low bioavailability of curcumin, which has been extensively reported in rodents and humans [20,21,22], is associated with a poor absorption, a high rate of metabolism, and a rapid excretion from the body. Studies conducted in rats after oral delivery, showed that most of the ingested curcumin is excreted in feces, which accounts for its weak bioavailability. Only small amounts are absorbed within the intestine and excreted in urine [22]. Pharmacokinetics studies conducted in rats showed that the oral bioavailability of curcumin is around 1% [23]. For instance, a maximum concentration (C_{max}) in the serum of only 500 ng/mL was reported after the oral delivery of 1 g/kg curcumin [24]. In another study, the C_{max} value after oral administration of 0.5 g/kg curcumin was 60 ng/mL, whereas a maximum serum concentration of 360 ng/mL was reached after i.v. delivery of 10 mg/kg curcumin [24]. In humans, a C_{max} value of 50 ng/mL was reported after oral administration of escalating doses from 500 mg to 12 g of curcumin [25]. However, while an oral dose of up to 8–12 g/day could be taken with no adverse effects [22], most of the clinical studies reported that the absorption and bioavailability of curcumin are very low since curcumin could not be detected in the serum of the majority of subjects [22]. This, in combination with the high degree of intestinal retention and retro-enteral efflux, translates to very low curcumin levels in tissue [14]. Distribution of curcumin through the body has been studied in rats where a strong variability in tissue distribution was reported [14,26,27]; however, because of the very low levels of curcumin observed in tissues, the relevance of these observations remain difficult to evaluate.

2.3. Curcumin Metabolism

Many studies have been carried out in rats and humans concerning curcumin metabolism, particularly in microsome fractions of intestinal or liver tissue homogenates. These studies have shown that curcumin metabolism mainly occurred via reduction followed by conjugation. Di-, tetra, hexa-, and octahydrocurcumin are the main degradation products resulting from reduction, which mainly occurs through the action of alcohol dehydrogenase [17,20,27,28,29]. Phase two metabolism, which occurs through glucuronidation/sulfonation conjugation, rapidly conjugates curcumin and its reduced metabolites [29,30,31,32]. Consequently, the small amount of curcumin that is absorbed by the body is found in the blood as glucuronide and sulfate metabolites [33].

2.4. Doses and Routes of Administration in PN Models

Despite its weak pharmacokinetics profile, numerous studies have reported a beneficial effect of curcumin on experimental models of PN, including peripheral nerve injury, hereditary PN (such as Charcot-Marie-Tooth (CMT) disease), alcohol-induced, chemotherapy-induced PN (CIPN), and diabetes-induced PN

(DPN). As shown in **Table 1**, in most of these studies, curcumin was delivered alone, preferentially through oral or intraperitoneal (i.p.) route, at dose ranging from 20 to 300 mg/kg/day and for 7 to 140 days. The use of high doses appears to be required in order to achieve systemic effect. Interestingly, when a local effect is sought, curcumin has also been shown to exert beneficial effects on peripheral nerve regeneration at very low concentrations [34]. Interestingly, in vitro studies show that curcumin at doses of 0.1 to 1 μM, stimulates the proliferation, migration, and lamellipod formation of Schwann cells, protects axons from degeneration induced by neuroinflammation, and reduces oxidative stress [34,35,36]. However, since the serum concentration after oral administration of curcumin is between 10 and 500 ng/ mL [22,23,24,25], the use of newer curcumin formulations to improve and better control the bioavailability of curcumin is essential.

Table 1

Summary of studies.

Experimental Model	Species	Delivery Method	Formulation	Dose (mg/ kg/ day)	References
Sciatic nerve crush	SD Rat	local (osmotic pumps), 28 days	Curcumin	0.2	[34]
Oxaliplatin-induced neuropathies	SD Rat	oral gavage, 28 days	Curcumin	12.5, 25, and 50	[39]
Oxaliplatin- and cisplatin-induced neuropathies	Wistar Rat	i.p., 32 days	Curcumin	10	[40]

Condition	Model	Route/Duration	Compound	Dose (mg/kg)	Ref
Cisplatin-induced neuropathy	Wistar Rat	oral, 35 days	Curcumin	200	[41]
Vincristine-induced neuropathy	Swiss Mouse	oral, 14 days	Curcumin	30 to 60	[42]
Vincristine-induced neuropathy	Wistar Rat	oral, 14 days	Tetrahydrocurcumin	40 and 80	[43]
Diabetic peripheral neuropathy	SD Rat	i.p., acute and chronic (days 7 to 21)	Curcumin	50	[44]
Diabetic peripheral neuropathy	Wistar Rat	oral, 6 weeks	Curcumin	50 or 100	[45]
Diabetic peripheral neuropathy	SD Rat	i.p., 14 days	Curcumin	200	[46]
Diabetic peripheral neuropathy	SD Rat	oral, 35 days	Curcumin	100	[47]
Diabetic peripheral neuropathy	SD Rat	oral, 28 days	Curcumin	60	[48]
Diabetic peripheral neuropathy	Laka Mouse	oral, 28 days	Curcumin	15 to 60	[49]
Diabetic peripheral neuropathy	SPF Rat	oral, 5 days	Curcumin derivative J147	10 to 100 μM	[50]
Diabetic peripheral neuropathy	SD Rat	oral, 14 days	Nano-emulsified curcumin	30 to 300	[51]
Diabetic	SD Rat	i.v., 2	Nanoparticle-	16	[52]

		injections (week 7 and 8)	encapsulated curcumin		
peripheral neuropathy					
Sciatic nerve chronic constriction injury	SD Rat	i.p., 7 days	Curcumin	20, 40 and 60	[53]
Postoperative pain (surgical paw incision)	SD Rat	p.o., acute	Curcumin	10 to 40	[54]
Sciatic nerve chronic constriction injury	SD Rat	oral, 7 days	Curcumin	50	[55]
Sciatic nerve chronic constriction injury	Wistar Rat	i.p., 1 week	Curcumin	12.5, 25, and 50	[56]
Sciatic nerve chronic constriction injury	C57BL /6J Mice	p.o., 3 weeks	Curcumin	5, 15 or 45	[57]
Spinal nerve ligation	Wistar Rat	Intrathecal and p.o.	Curcumin	i.t. 30 to 300 μg / p.o. 10 to 310	[58]
Sciatic nerve section	BALB/ c Mouse	i.p., twice daily for 7 days	Curcumin	30 to 120 mg/kg	[59]
Brachial plexus avulsion	SD Rat	i.p., 28 days	Curcumin	60	[60]
Alcohol-induced neuropathy	Wistar Rat	oral, 70 days	Curcumin	20 to 80	[61]

Alcohol-induced neuropathy	Wistar Rat	i.p., 63 days	Curcumin	60	[62]
Opioid-induced hyperalgesia	C57BL /6J Mice	i.p., 6 days	Curcumin	50	[63]
HIV-gp120-induced neuropathic pain	SD Rat	i.v., 3 injections (days 7, 10 and 13)	Nanoparticle-encapsulated curcumin	4	[64]
Complete Freund's adjuvant induced neuropathic pain	Charles-Foster Rat	i.p., acute	Curcumin	100	[65]
Sciatic nerve crush in diabetic condition	SD Rat	i.p., 28 days	Curcumin	50 to 300	[66]
Diabetic peripheral neuropathy	Swiss Mouse	oral gavage, twice daily 20 weeks	Curcumin derivative J147	10 to 50	[67]
Sciatic nerve crush	Wistar Rat	oral, 28 days	Curcumin	100	[68]
Sciatic nerve excision	Wistar Rat	local (nerve conducts)	Curcumin	10 μL at 5 mg/ mL	[69]
Hereditary peripheral neuropahty (CMT1A)	Mouse (*Tr-J*)	oral, 90 days	Curcumin	100	[70]
Hereditary peripheral neuropahty	Mouse (*Tr-J*)	oral, 90 days	Curcumin	100	[71]

(CMT1A)					
Hereditary peripheral neuropahty (CMT1A)	Rat SD (*PMP22*)	i.p., 8 weeks	Curcumin–cyclodextrin/cellulose Nanocrystals	0.2	[72]
Hereditary peripheral neuropahty (CMT1B)	Mouse (R98C)	oral, 39 days	Curcumin	100	[73]
Sciatic nerve amputation	BALB/c Mouse	oral, 7 days	Curcumin	20 to 40	[74]
Sciatic nerve chronic constriction injury	SD Rat	i.p., 14 days	Curcumin	100	[75]
Sciatic nerve crush	SD Rat	oral, 28 days	Curcumin	100	[76]
Sciatic nerve crush	Wistar Rat	i.p., 4 weeks	Curcumin	100	[77]
Sciatic nerve crush	SD Rat	i.p., 28 days	Curcumin	100	[78]
Sciatic nerve crush	SD Rat	i.p., 60 days	Curcumin	100	[79]
Sciatic nerve transection	Wistar Rat	i.p., 28 days	Curcumin	100	[80]

Open in a separate window

2.5. New Curcumin Formulations

Recently, chemical modifications of curcumin and the development of various types of biopolymers used as carriers were shown to improve the solubility, the bioavailability, and the pharmacokinetics profile of curcumin [37,38]. However, although these new curcumin formulations allow the use of lower doses (that are compatible with clinical application), to date, only few of these formulations have been studied in the context of PN (Table

1).

3. Curcumin Studies in Animal Models of PN

3.1. Behavioral Aspects

The neuropathy models, curcumin doses, routes of administration, and species of animals in the various studies are summarized in **Table 1**.

3.1.1. Neuropathic Pain The symptomatology of PN is very diverse depending notably of the ethology. Neuropathic pain and hypersensitivity are reported in chronic constriction injury, nerve ligature, brachial plexus avulsion, diabetic, alcohol, and CIPN. The tests used to measure pain-related behaviors in animal models of neuropathies are hot/cold-plate, tail-flick immersion, Hargreaves and acetone tests for cold and thermal hypersensitivity. Von Frey filaments, pin prick, and Randall-Selitto tests are, for their part, used to measure mechanical hypersensitivity. Numerous studies have shown that curcumin and its derivatives have an antinociceptive effect by decreasing mechanical, thermal, and cold hypersensitivity in PN models. For example, curcumin, using oral or i.p. injections, decreased mechanical, thermal, and cold hypersensitivity in three models of CIPN (oxaliplatin, vincristine, and cisplatin) on male Sprague Dawley (SD) rats [39], on male Wistar rats [40,41] and on male Swiss albino mice [42]. In addition, tetrahydrocurcumin, a major metabolite of curcumin (see above), significantly decreased vincristine-induced hypersensitivity in male Wistar rats, measured via hot/cold plate and Randall-Selitto tests [43]. The antinociceptive properties of curcumin and its derivatives have also been reported in models of streptozotocin (STZ)-induced DPN. Curcumin reduced mechanical, cold, and thermal hypersensitivity in male Wistar and SD rats [44,45,46,47,48] and male Laka albino mouse models of DPN obtained by injection of STZ [49]. New formulations of curcumin have also shown an antinociceptive effect on mechanical, cold, and thermal hypersensitivity in models of DPN with sometimes superior effects to unformulated curcumin. For example, Ly et al. 2018, showed in male SPF rats that curcumin J147 (hybrid molecule between curcumin and cyclohexyl-bisphenol-A) decreased STZ-induced mechanical hypersensitivity in the von Frey test [50]. In addition, an alternative curcumin delivery system, self-nano-emulsifying drug delivery system (SNEDDS) curcumin, reversed, in male SD rat model of DPN, the mechanical hypersensitivity to hot and cold measured by von Frey test and tail flick hot and cold immersions, respectively [51]. Nanoparticle-encapsulated curcumin (curcumin-polybutylcyanoacrylate nanoparticle-encapsulated particles: PEGMA-DMAEMA-MAO) has also been investigated in DPN male SD rat model and showed a reduction of both thermal and mechanical hypersensitivity [52]. Other models widely used in the study of neuropathic pain are the chronic constriction injury (CCI) and nerve ligature models. In these models, animals develop chronic inflammatory pain. Thus, in particular by its anti-inflammatory action, curcumin reduced mechanical and thermal hypersensitivity in the CCI model in SD rats [53,54,55], in Wistar rats [56], in male C57BL/6J mice [57], and in nerve ligature model in female Wistar rats [58] and in BALB/c mice [59]. Finally, curcumin also showed antinociceptive properties in SD rats in models of brachial plexus avulsion [60], alcohol-induced neuropathy in male and female Wistar rats [61,62], opioid-induced hyperalgesia in C57-BL/6J mice [63], HIV-gp120-induced neuropathic pain in male SD rats [64], and complete Freund's adjuvant-induced inflammatory pain in Charles-Foster strain rats [65].

While the use of different doses, curcumin derivatives, rodent species and strains made comparisons between studies difficult, the results show clearly that curcumin possesses antinociceptive properties in various animal models of PN. However, the majority of these studies used evoked responses (reflexive tests) as pain-related measures and no spontaneous pain assessments were reported.

3.1.2. Loss of Sensitivity A number of PN do not present pain but, on the contrary, loss of sensitivity. This is particularly the case in pathologies of genetic origin (CMT for example) or of traumatic origin (nerve crushing and transection). In this case, the substantial loss of sensory nerve fibers leads to loss of sensitivity. This loss or decrease in sensitivity can be measured in animal models by the same tests as described above. For example, curcumin, because of its neuro-protective effects, has shown to improve mechanical and thermal sensitivity in models of sciatic nerve crushing. In a first study, curcumin was administered locally as close as possible to the lesion site (with an osmotic mini pump) and showed a faster recovery of mechanical sensitivity as measured by the von Frey test in male SD rats [34]. A second study, also conducted in a male SD rat sciatic nerve crush model, showed a faster recovery of mechanical and thermal sensitivity after i.p. injection of curcumin and was dose-dependent [66].

3.1.3. Motor Dysfunctions Finally, if the motor nerve fibers are damaged (which is the case in many neuropathies), there is a loss of contact with the muscle fibers and thus motor dysfunctions. Motor behavior is thus studied in animals by various tests such as, locomotor activity by activity meter test, locomotor coordination by rotarod test, walking track analyze by sciatic function index (SFI), finger spacing by visual static sciatic index (SSI), muscular strength by grip strength test, and skilled locomotion by beam walking test. Curcumin, because of its neuro-protective effect and its ability to stimulate axonal regrowth, has shown to significantly improve motor function in various models of PN. Thus, it has been reported that curcumin improved locomotor activity in both cisplatin- and oxaliplatin-induced neuropathies in Wistar rats [40]. In addition, curcumin and tetrahydrocurcumin improved the SFI score and locomotor coordination in a vincristine-induced PN, in male swiss mouse and Wistar rat respectively [42,43]. Curcumin also allowed a faster recovery of locomotor activity in CCI model [54], of locomotor coordination in alcohol-induced neuropathy [62] and in DPN models [67]. Curcumin improved locomotor coordination, walking track analysis, finger spacing, muscular strength, and skilled locomotion in traumatic neuropathies induced by sciatic nerve crush or transection in male SD rats [34,66], in female Wistar rats [68], and in male Wistar rats [69]. Finally, locomotor coordination and muscle strength were significantly improved in CMT1A mouse model (*Trembler*-J mice C57BL/6J) [70,71], CMT1A rat model (PMP22, SD) [72] and CMT1B mouse model (heterozygous R98C mice) [73]. For example, in CMT1B model, overexpression of the myelin protein myelin protein zero (MPZ), which induces cytotoxicity in Schwann cells (SCs) and thus locomotor dysfunction, was reduced by the anti-ER-stress effect of curcumin [73].

3.2. Electrophysiology Aspects

Electrophysiological measurements are an important component in the assessment of PN. These are easily comparable measurements between animals and humans. These measurements are in the majority of cases performed on the caudal nerve of the animal's tail or by exposing the sciatic nerve. Two main parameters are measured, nerve conduction velocity and signal amplitude. The reduction in nerve conduction velocity is closely related to a reduction in the thickness of the myelin sheath, while the reduction in signal amplitude corresponds to a reduction in the number of nerve fibers. It has been shown that because of its lipophilic character, curcumin is easily and stably inserted into the lipid bilayers of the myelin sheath and thus can have a protective effect on the myelin sheath thus improving nerve conduction [34]. Curcumin has been shown to improve the electrophysiological parameters in three CIPN models. For example, Zhang et al. 2020 showed in male SD rats that the decrease in motor nerve conduction velocity (MNCV) and sensory nerve conduction velocity (SNCV) observed after oxaliplatin injection were both increased after curcumin administration and were dose-dependent [39]. In addition, curcumin reverses the reduction of MNCV in the cisplatin model in female Wistar rats [41]. Similarly, tetrahydrocurcumin also restored MNCV in a vincristine-induced neuropathy model in male Wistar rats [43]. Curcumin has also shown beneficial effects on electrophysiological parameters in other chronic inflammatory neuropathies such as diabetes and alcohol. For example, two formulations of curcumin J147 and SNEDDS improved MNCV in models of DPN in female Swiss mice [67] and in male SD rats [51] and curcumin improved MNCV in ethanol-induced neuropathy model in male and female Wistar rats [61]. Finally, in models of traumatic and genetic neuropathies, in which nerve fibers and the myelin sheath are damaged, curcumin improved nerve conduction velocity and amplitude. Indeed, whether in models of sciatic nerve crush in female Wistar rats [68] and in male SD rats [34,66] or in models of complete nerve transection in BALB/c mice [74], curcumin allowed faster recovery of electrophysiological parameters, such as increased nerve conduction velocity and signal amplitude. Finally, compound muscle action potential amplitudes were also increased by curcumin treatment in a model of demyelinating neuropathy of genetic origin in CMT1A rats [72] and R98C mice (CMT1B) [73].

3.3. Histological Aspects

The sites of action of curcumin in peripheral neuropathies as reported in the literature are summarized in Figure 1.

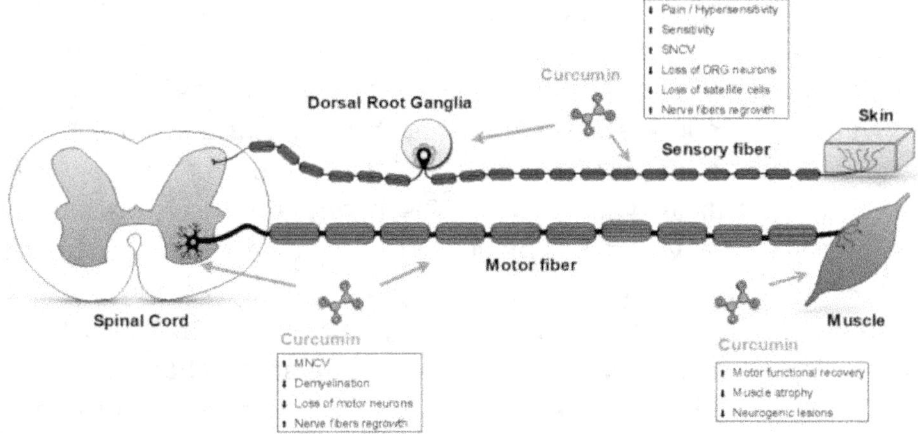

Figure 1

A suggested model summarizing the sites of action of curcumin in peripheral neuropathies as reported in the literature: curcumin reduces neuropathic pain and improves sensitivity in in vivo models of PN, by improving sensory nerve conduction velocity (SNCV), reducing the loss of neurons and satellite cells in dorsal roots ganglia (DRG), and promoting the regrowth of sensory nerve fibers. In addition, curcumin improves motor functions in in vivo models of PN, by improving motor nerve conduction velocity (MNCV), reducing nerve fibers demyelination, loss of motor neurons in spinal cord, muscle atrophy and neurogenic lesions, and improving motor nerves fibers regrowth.

3.3.1. Nerve Fibers and Myelin

PN primarily affect the nerves and notably result in a degeneration of the axons, known as Wallerian degeneration, and in a demyelination of these same axons. In some neuropathies only the axons are affected and in others only the myelin sheath. However, in the majority of cases both axons and myelin are affected. In the study published by Caillaud et al. 2018, curcumin increased the expression of myelin protein zero and myelin basic protein 22, and the thickness of the myelin sheath, and decreased neurogenic lesions of the sciatic nerve [34]. In spite of the differences in the route of administration, Ma et al. 2013 showed similar results where daily i.p. injections of 100 and 300 mg/kg of curcumin for 4 weeks promoted faster nerve regeneration after peripheral nerve injury [66]. Similar outcomes were found in a complete amputation of sciatic nerve in Balb/c mice. Intragastrical administration of 20 and 40 mg/kg/day curcumin for 1 week positively affected nerve regeneration and functional recovery in 8 weeks post-surgery. Histological analysis showed dose-dependent myelin sheath thickening with 40 mg/kg/day being the more effective in reversing damage to the nerve [74]. Rats that underwent CCI or CCI-chronic constriction release of the sciatic nerve also showed after curcumin oral treatment greater axonal regeneration and weaker degeneration of nerve tissues [75]. In hereditary neuropathy models of CMT, a 90-day curcumin treatment by oral gavage starting at postnatal day 4 in R98C CMT1B and Tremble-J mice, and i.p. injection in CMT1A rats, increased the number of large-diameter axons, higher average of fibers, axonal size, and myelin thickness in the sciatic nerve [71,72,73]. Nerve fiber degeneration and swelling, wide endoneurial space, disrupted myelin sheath, as well as swelling of SCs are histological markers of alcohol-induced neuropathy in rats. Administration of 60 mg/kg curcumin decreased these effects and also had a regenerative effect on the nerve fibers in the sciatic nerve [62]. Likewise, male rats concomitantly treated with chemotherapeutic drugs, such as cisplatin and oxaliplatin, and curcumin showed improvements in functional outcome and myelin loss by decreasing demyelination [40]. Tetrahydrocurcumin, had a dose-dependent protective action against nerve damage and axonal swelling. The higher dose of tetrahydrocurcumin (80 mg/kg) showed a better neuroprotective activity than the 40 mg/kg, with no axonal swelling of the sciatic nerve [43].

3.3.2. DRGs and Spinal Cord Neurons The dorsal root ganglia (DRG) are active participants that relay signaling from the periphery to the central nervous system [81]. Therefore, it is not a surprise to find pathological changes in these DRG in PN. For example, morphological changes in the DRG were observed in rat sciatic nerve crush model in particular on the neuronal population type A and B and satellite cells. The addition of curcumin showed a 17% type A and 36% type B cells increase compared to the untreated sciatic nerve crush group. Satellite cells (glial cells that cover the surface of DRG neurons) also showed a decrease after sciatic nerve crush and the curcumin-treated group showed a 19% increase in satellite cells compared to the untreated sciatic nerve crush group [76]. The impact of CCI in DRGs includes vacuolization, increase in the sizes of cells due to swelling, and loss of nuclei. These changes partially decreased in the curcumin-treated animals [75]. Morphometric analysis of DRGs from cisplatin-treated rats revealed a significant atrophy of the nuclei and nucleoli. When treated with curcumin (200 mg/kg/day by gavage, 5 weeks), the nucleolar atrophy was prevented, and the nuclear atrophy was partially blocked. Curcumin was also found to partially reduce the loss of DRG neurons [41]. While CIPN primary targets mainly involve peripheral nerves, recent data suggest direct toxicity in spinal cord neurons [82]. The functional state of neuronal cells can be assessed by formational changes in the Nissl bodies [83]. Spinal cord analysis of rats subjected to oxaliplatin showed curcumin-induced repairs injury in the spinal dorsal horn. Treatment with curcumin, 12.5, 25, or 50 mg/kg by gavage for 28 consecutive days, showed neatly arranged neurons that had wide intercellular space and a small number of Nissl bodies compared to the negative control. The higher dose of curcumin showed organized neurons with compact intercellular spacing and no Nissl body fragmentation [39].

3.3.3. Muscles Denervation of the gastrocnemius muscles leads to muscle neurogenic lesions seen as clusters of small skeletal muscle fibers with central nuclei. General muscle atrophy can also be reported because of a decrease in the size of muscle fibers. Caillaud et al. 2018 reported that local delivery of curcumin (0.25 µL/h) via a mini osmotic pump for five weeks post sciatic nerve crush improved the diameter of muscle fibers of rats.

In addition, this study showed positive effect of curcumin on gastrocnemius muscle fibers repartition limiting the presence of clusters of small skeletal muscle fibers [34]. In another study on nerve crush injury model, rats treated with curcumin showed a motor functional recovery and reversal of gastrocnemius muscle atrophy after four weeks of daily treatment post-surgery. The recovery rate was dose-specific where groups treated with more potent curcumin solutions (100 mg/kg or 300 mg/kg) showed a significant increase in the average of muscle fiber area as compared to the vehicle and 50 mg/kg-treated group. All three doses of curcumin enhanced motoneurons regeneration which was concluded by a significantly higher number of myelinated axons per nerve transverse section and a higher mean diameter of nerve fibers than that in the vehicle group [66]. Similar results were observed by another group in a sciatic nerve crush in rats. Rodents administered with daily 100 mg/kg of curcumin (i.p.) for 4 weeks after the surgery presented smaller extent of gastrocnemius muscle atrophy, measured as muscle weight; and larger muscle diameter when compared to sham and vehicle-treated groups [77].

4. Curcumin Mechanisms of Action and Cellular Targets in the Treatment of PN

The molecular targets of curcumin in peripheral neuropathies reported in the literature are summarized in Figure 2.

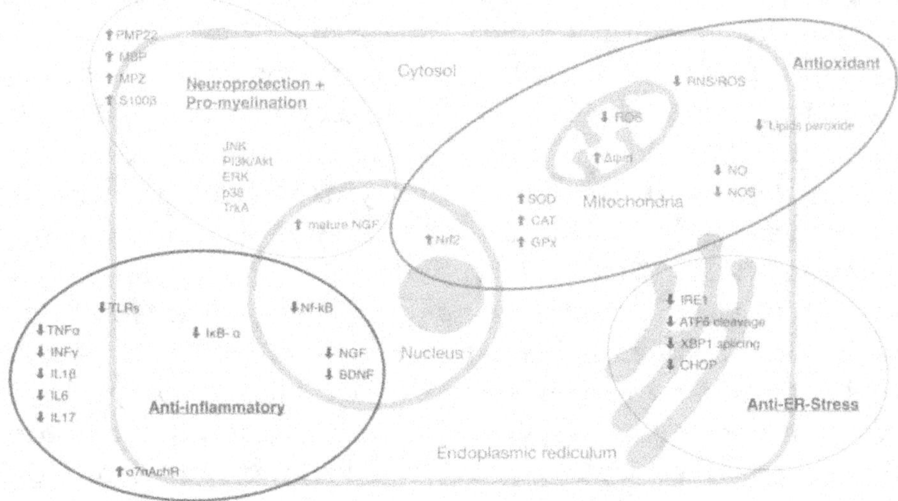

Figure 2

A proposed model summarizing the molecular targets of curcumin in peripheral neuropathies reported in the literature: tumor necrosis factors (TNFα), interferon (INF-γ), interleukins (IL-1α, IL-1β, IL-6, IL_10), granulocyte-macrophage colony-stimulating factor (GM-CSF), monocyte chemoattractant protein-1 (MCP-1), and macrophage inflammatory protein (MIP-1α), Toll-like receptor (TLR, TLR1, TLR3, TLR4, and TLR7), nuclear factor-kappa B (NF-κB), NF-κB inhibitor-α (IκB-α), nerve growth factor (NGF), brain derived neurotrophic factor (BDNF), lipooxygenase (LOX), cyclooxygenase (COX), nitric oxide synthase (NOS), superoxide dismutase (SOD), catalase (CAT), glutathione peroxidase (GPx), transient receptor potential cation channel subfamily-M-2 (TRMP2), nuclear factor erythroid 2–related factor 2 (Nrf2), reactive oxygen species (ROS), reactive nitrogen species (RNS), peripheral myelin protein 22 (PMP22), myelin protein zero (MPZ), myelin basic protein (MBP), extracellular signal regulated kinase (ERK), c-Jun-N-terminal kinase (JNK), α7-nicotinic acetylcholine receptors (α7-nAchR), tropomyosin receptor kinase A (TrkA), phosphoinositide 3-kinase (PI3K), activating transcription factor 3 (ATF3), ER-residing protein endoplasmic oxidoreductin-1 (Ero-1β), activating transcription factor 6 (ATF6) cleavage, X-Box binding protein 1 (XBP1) splicing, and C/EBP homologous protein (CHOP).

4.1. Curcumin's Anti-Inflammatory Properties

Chronic or acute inflammation is a physiological process present in all PN with a preponderance in DPN, CIPN, toxic, and traumatic neuropathies. For example, nerve damage in the peripheral nervous system has been previously established to induce Wallerian degeneration, a highly inflammatory response in which

SCs that dissociate from damaged axons release cytokines such as tumor necrosis factors (TNFα), interferon (INF-γ), interleukins (IL-1α, IL-1β, IL-6, IL_10), granulocyte-macrophage colony-stimulating factor (GM-CSF), monocyte chemoattractant protein-1 (MCP-1), and macrophage inflammatory protein (MIP-1α) [84]. Upon dissociation, this cytokine release is mediated by an increase in SCs of Toll-like receptor (TLR) expression, specifically TLR1, TLR3, TLR4, and TLR7 which bind to both endogenous and exogenous ligands [85]. The downstream effect is the activation of nuclear factor-kappa B (NF-κB) [86], the release of cytokines and the recruitment of macrophages, lymphocytes, neutrophils and mast cells, which further increases inflammation [85]. The type of leukocyte recruited varies across different pathologies and mediates symptoms of PN. One of curcumin's beneficial properties is its anti-inflammatory effects. In in vitro studies, it decreases the activation of NF-κB downstream of TLRs by decreasing the phosphorylation of its regulator, NF-κB inhibitor-α (IκB-α) [86]. Unphosphorylated IκB-α binds to NF-κB and prevents its translocation to the nucleus, thus inhibiting downstream expression and release of cytokines [86]. Similarly, in vivo studies have shown curcumin to dose-dependently downregulate the expression of INF-γ [87], TNF-α [39,43,60,61,67,87,88], IL-1β [39,61,87], IL-17 [87], IL-6 [39,61,87], and C-reactive protein [67]. This downregulation of cytokines is seen systemically in the sciatic nerve, whole brain, and spinal cord samples of autoimmune neuritis, alcoholic neuropathy, sciatic nerve injury, chemotherapy-induced peripheral neurotoxicity, and various rodent models used in the studies above. Nerve growth factor (NGF), c-Fos [60], brain-derived neurotrophic factor (BDNF) [53], and Cox-2 [53] are some markers for inflammation-mediated pain [60]. As curcumin has the capacity to reduce the inflammatory response, spinal cord expression of both NGF and c-Fos was reduced in a brachial plexus avulsion model [60]. The assumption is that the NGF measured was pro-NGF, since this is the form of NGF involved in neuronal apoptosis and death [78]. p300 and CREB-binding protein (CBP) histone acetyl transferases (HATs) mediate the expression of the other two markers, BDNF and Cox-2 [53]. Chronic constriction injury models treated with curcumin had reduced promoter acetylation and subsequent reduced expression of BDNF and Cox-2 in the spinal cord [53]. The decrease in expression paired with behavioral findings of lower threshold for mechanical, heat, and cold allodynia provides support for curcumin's anti-nociceptive effects via its anti-inflammatory pathways [53,60].

4.2. Curcumin Reduces Oxidative Stress

Oxidative stress and inflammation are closely related pathophysiological processes, one of which can be easily induced by the other. Hence, when peripheral nerve damage induces an inflammatory response, oxidative stress will also be activated. Oxidative stress encompasses the production of reactive oxygen and nitrogen species (ROS/RNS) such as hydrogen peroxide, superoxide radicals, hydroxyl radicals, and nitric oxide radicals which imposes cellular damage [87]. Lipooxygenase (LOX), cyclooxygenase (COX), and nitric oxide synthase (NOS) play major roles in their production while superoxide dismutase (SOD), catalase (CAT), and glutathione peroxidase (GPx) are involved in their elimination [89]. Curcumin decreased lipid peroxide [34,39,42,43,61,62], nitrite [61], NOS [67], and NO [42,43] levels. In the optic nerve, ROS has been reported to activate transient receptor potential channels, especially transient receptor potential cation channel subfamily-M-2 (TRMP2), which causes an influx of Ca_{2+}, thus mediating nerve damage [90]. TRMP2 activation was reduced with curcumin, resulting in decreased mitochondrial membrane depolarization and further decrease in the production of reactive oxygen species (ROS) and reactive nitrogen species (RNS) [90].

Antioxidative mechanisms are also upregulated by curcumin treatment. Nuclear factor erythroid 2–related factor 2 (Nrf2), a transcription factor which activates the antioxidant response element (ARE), is upregulated with curcumin [34]. The downstream effect of ARE activation is the production of antioxidative enzymes, and accordingly, curcumin was reported to increase SOD [39,42,43,86], CAT [39,42,43,86], and GPx [42,43] activity. This increase was observed in the sciatic nerve and cortical neurons of in vivo experimental rodent models of CIPN. Taken together, curcumin has the ability to: (i) Decrease the production of total and mitochondrial ROS/RNS; (ii) decrease lipoperoxidation of membrane lipids; and (iii) increase levels of antioxidant enzymes (SOD, CAT, GPx) mediated by transcription factor Nrf2.

4.3. Curcumin Relieves Endoplasmic Reticulum (ER) Stress

A growing body of evidence shows a strong link between oxidative stress and ER stress in neurological diseases [91]. Indeed, the ER redox environment dictates the fate of entering proteins in ER [91]. Thus, an increase in intracellular oxidative stress is unfavorable to the proper folding of proteins. Protein misfolding and ER stress have been commonly reported in PN, such as CMT disease [73,92]. CMT disease is the most common inheritable PN with various subtypes (CMT1, CMT2, DI-CMT, CMT4, and CMTX…) [2]. Of these, CMT1, especially CMT1A and CMT1B, involves demyelination of peripheral nerves [2]. CMT1A and CMT1B are caused by mutations in peripheral myelin protein 22 (PMP22) [72] and myelin protein zero (MPZ) respectively, resulting in misfolded protein accumulation in the ER of SCs [93]. This accumulation activates the unfolded protein response (UPR) which causes ER stress, oxidative stress, and subsequent apoptosis of SCs [94]. Curcumin dose-dependently decreased the accumulation of mutant proteins in the ER [92], apoptosis rate [70,92], UPR markers activating transcription factor 3 (ATF3), ER-residing protein endoplasmic oxidoreductin-1 (Ero-1β) [71], activating transcription factor 6 (ATF6) cleavage, X-Box binding protein 1 (XBP1) splicing, and C/EBP homologous protein (CHOP) [73]. The effect of curcumin on Chop expression remains unclear as no effect was observed in Okamoto et al.'s 2013 study while in Patzko Bai et al.'s 2012 study a decrease in Chop was seen that did not undergo nuclear translocation [71,73]. In addition, a limitation of these studies is the use of HeLa and HEK293 cells, very far from the SC phenotype. Nevertheless, the hypothesized mechanism of action for curcumin's ER stress relief is proposed to be through the modulation of ER calcium levels, impairing calcium-dependent chaperones (calnexin, calreticulin) and subsequently decreasing the UPR or activation of endoplasmic-reticulum-associated protein degradation (ERAD) pathway [72,73,92]. Additionally, the expression of heat shock protein 70 (Hsp70) appears to be an important factor in curcumin's UPR reduction [71,72].

4.4. Curcumin Recruits Schwann Cells, Induces Remyelination and Nerve Regeneration

Peripheral nerve demyelination develops in conditions such Guillain-Barre syndrome (GBS), chronic inflammatory demyelinating polyradiculoneuropathy (CIDP), paraneoplastic neuropathy, CMT, vitamin deficiencies, and CIPN [2]. Demyelination can be mediated through various mechanisms, from autoimmunity (CIDP) to SC dissociation from axons, SC apoptosis, oxidative stress, and inflammation [95]. Myelination by SCs is mediated by the NF-κB pathway, wherein axons and laminin induce the phosphorylation of p65 which activates NF-κB, a pro-myelinating transcription factor as seen above [35,73]. Curcumin induces remyelination by increasing NF-κB levels [35] and by increasing MPZ [34], PMP22 [34,79], S100β [69,74,77,79], and MBP levels [35,79]. These markers are indicative of increased SC recruitment and promyelinating activity. As such, an increase in myelin thickness [34,40,41,66,69,70,76,80] and axon diameter [34,66,70,74,76,80] is observed with curcumin treatment. Also, of note is the proposed involvement of extracellular signal-regulated kinase (ERK) and p38 kinases [35]. The former promotes myelination and the latter the opposite. Accordingly, treatment with curcumin yielded an increase in ERK and a decrease in phosphorylated p38 [35] in SC cultures, providing more evidence for its remyelination properties. Demyelination upon insult is typically followed by axonal degeneration and this can be mediated by the activation of the microglial TLR-4/My88 and axonal c-Jun-N-terminal kinase (JNK) pathways [36]. Curcumin interferes with the JNK pathway in axons to exert its neuroprotective effects [36,66,69], in both in vitro (hippocampal neurons) and in vivo models of sciatic nerve transection and sciatic nerve crush injury. Similarly, curcumin downregulates JNK and upregulates promyelinating Krox-20 expression in SCs in CMT 1B model [73]. In PN such as CIPN, the effects are not limited to the extremities and can affect the DRG. This is reflected in the reduction in neuronal size/volume and the number of DRG neuronal population [41,76]. Curcumin's effects are systematic as they increased DRG neuron size and population in CIPN and in sciatic nerve crush models [41,76], with the proposed mechanism being via curcumin's antioxidative properties [41]. Some other ways of assessing nerve regeneration are by looking at nerve fibers regrowth and functional recovery. As seen in the DRG, after curcumin treatment, the number of sciatic nerve fiber increased [66,69,74,80] in rodent models of sciatic nerve transection, nerve crush injury, and even complete sciatic nerve amputation. The sciatic functional index (SFI) also improved in the above models [66,69,76]. NGF, particularly mature NGF, has also been implicated in regenerative pathways. NGF binds to tropomyosin receptor kinase A (TrkA) and p57 receptors, with mature NGF binding to the former and pro NGF to the latter [78]. As such, TrkA is involved in protective and regenerative pathways while p57 is involved in apoptosis [78]. Downstream of TrkA is the activation of phosphoinositide 3-kinase (PI3K)/Akt pathway, which inhibits mitochondrial damage and thus cell death [78]. In both in vitro (PC12 cell line) and in vivo studies, curcumin increased TrkA, Akt, and mature NGF levels while decreasing pro NGF and caspase 3 levels, resulting in apoptotic reduction. Curcumin therefore has the capacity to promote remyelination and regeneration through modulation of the NF-κB, JNK and PI3K/Akt pathways. However, more work needs to be conducted to unravel curcumin's regenerative mechanisms as it is not as well understood as remyelination.

Interestingly, an in vitro study shows that curcumin at low doses stimulates the proliferation, migration and lamellipod formation of SCs [35]. In addition, curcumin have been shown to protect axons from degeneration induced by local neuroinflammation in vitro [36]. In addition, low concentrations of curcumin stimulate the proliferation of embryonic neuronal progenitor cells in vitro [96]. Another in vitro study on neurite outgrowth inhibition in PC12 by cisplatin showed reduction of cisplatin-induced inhibition of neurite outgrowth by up to 50% with curcumin treatment [97]. Finally, curcumin has also been reported in vitro to act as a type II positive allosteric modulator of α7-nicotinic acetylcholine receptors (α7-nAchR), decreasing their desensitization and even promoting reactivation of the desensitized pool in Xenopus oocytes expression human receptors [98]. This translates into decreased nociception (reduced acetic acid-induced stretching and reduced paw licking with plantar formalin injection) in in vivo studies and the same therapeutic mechanism has been postulated for curcumin's effect on microglia [98].

5. Curcumin in Clinical Studies for PN

Because of the abundant amount of preclinical data showing the antioxidant and anti-inflammatory properties of curcuminoids, most clinical studies using curcumin have investigated its therapeutic effects in patient diagnosed with chronic inflammatory joint pain, such as osteoarthritis and rheumatoid arthritis. In many of the most recent randomized clinical trials, patients received various formulations of oral curcumin which were designed to enhance its bioavailability compared to the traditional powered extract, such as BCM-95 ®, Theracurmin ® and

Meriva ®. BCM-95 ® and Theracurmin® were shown to reduce knee pain scores respectively in patients with rheumatoid arthritis [99] and osteoarthritis [100]. Meriva® was able to reduce knee pain and blood plasma levels of the inflammatory markers IL-β1 and IL-6 in patients with osteoarthritis [101].

However, clinical studies showing curcumin efficacy in patients diagnosed with PN are substantially lacking. Di Piero et al. (2013) [102] studied the impact of curcumin on chronic neuropathic pain in patients diagnosed with lumbar disc herniation and/or lumbar canal stenosis or carpal tunnel syndrome. Patients were segregated into one of three groups where they received Seractil (dexibuprofen 400 mg/tablet, twice/day), Seractil plus Tiobec 400 (lipoic acid 400 mg/tablet, twice/day), or Seractil plus Lipicur (400 mg lipoic acid with 400 mg curcumin and 4 mg piperine) for 8 weeks. The addition of curcumin to dexibuprofen and lipoic acid regimen significantly reduced neuropathic pain scores in both carpal tunnel and lumbar sciatica patients at 8 weeks post intervention. Curcumin was also shown to reduce the use of dexibuprofen by almost 3 weeks in these patients. Although these results seem promising for the therapeutic use of curcumin in patients with chronic neuropathy, it is impossible to distinguish if these beneficial effects are the result of the bioactive properties of curcumin or coactivity with lipoic acid.

In another observational study by Belcaro et al. 2013 [103], 80 cancer patients undergoing chemotherapy treatment orally received either one tablet of Meriva® 500 mg/day or a placebo for four months. Patients in the Meriva ® group self-reported significantly lower incidence of side effects from chemotherapy, which was further confirmed via semi-quantitative evaluation of cancer chemotherapy side effects, compared to those in the control group. Additionally, plasma free radical levels at the end of the study were observed to be reduced from levels at inclusion in patients given Meriva, while free radical levels increased in the control group.

Asadi et al. 2019 [104] led an 8-week double-blind randomized clinical trial that enrolled 80 patients with type 2 diabetes mellitus. Patients were diagnosed with diabetic peripheral neuropathy via Toronto Clinical Neuropathy Score (TCNS), with a blinded neurologist performing the clinical assessments before and after treatment. Patients were segregated into two groups which received either a polysorbate 80 placebo or an 80 mg nano-curcumin supplement composed of 72% curcumin, 25% desmethoxycurcumin, and 3% bisdemethoxycurcumin. Patients in the curcumin group self-reported a significant decrease in the mean scores of depression and anxiety, assessed via DASS-21-items questionnaire, 8 weeks post treatment. However, when the clinicians compared patient TCNS results, they did not observe any significant differences in the severity of neuropathy at inclusion or 8 weeks post treatment between the curcumin and placebo groups.

A case study by Burns et al. 2009 [105] focused on a 15-year-old, Caucasian, female diagnosed with Déjérine-Sottas disease, a hereditary neurological disorder characterized by damage to the peripheral nerves and resulting in progressive muscle wasting, who was given non-formulated, powdered curcumin in capsules for 12 months as a potential therapeutic regimen for her PN. The patient orally administered 50 mg/kg/day of curcumin (6 × 250 mg capsules three times/day, 1500 mg total) for the first 4 months, and then 75 mg/kg/day (10 × 250 mg capsules three times/day, 2500 mg total) for the remaining 8 months of this 12-month study. After the treatment, the patient displayed no adverse effects but little or no improvement in outcome measures such as muscle strength and upper/lower extremity disability. Similarly, the patient's neurophysiologic findings were unchanged after 12 months of curcumin treatment. The authors suggested that the patient may not have improved because of her neuropathy possibly having progressed to a point where the potential for recovery was limited, the efficacy of curcumin in patients with Déjérine-Sottas disease may be mutation-dependent, doses used may have been inadequate, or that the dose period may have been too short.

As described above, there is promising data to show that curcumin may have merit in alleviating some aspects of neuropathy in various patient populations, however, more clinical studies are needed in order to fully discern the safety and efficacy of curcumin administration in patients diagnosed with PN. Clinical studies using curcumin and its various formulations have shown that these drugs demonstrate a safety profile and have efficacious effects when used to treat patients diagnosed with chronic inflammatory joint pains. Finally, curcumin have anti-tumor effect and so would be a good drug candidate for CIPN treatment (no concerns by oncologists or patients about adverse effects and tumor growth) [106].

6. Conclusions

Curcumin is a lipophilic molecule that is rapidly metabolized, leading to low bioavailability. Thus, several studies propose the use of new formulations of curcumin such as emulsions or nanoparticles to improve systemic bioavailability. These approaches are very interesting in the context of several PN in which nerves are affected (diabetes, alcohol, chemotherapy, genetic mutations...). Moreover, these approaches allow to decrease and better control the dose of curcumin used, although it has no proven toxicity. In this respect, there is growing evidence that curcumin nanoparticles have a better effect on oxidative stress than conventional curcumin. Other authors propose in the case of localized lesions, as in the case of traumatic lesion, transection or local inflammation, the use of biofunctionalized conduit with curcumin or local administration at the site of the lesion. Thus, the use of these new approaches (nanoparticles, tubes...) allows a progressive diffusion of curcumin in the target organism or organ. This makes it possible to avoid the "one shot" effect produced by a conventional injection. This diffusion is all the more interesting as it allows a better reduction of inflammation and oxidative stress, which are processes that last over time and can be chronic. Thus, curcumin because of its anti-inflammatory, antioxidant, anti-ER-stress, and neuro-protective properties is the perfect candidate for the treatment of PN. In addition, its lipophilic nature allows it to be integrated into the myelin sheath, thus exerting a powerful antioxidant effect. The role of curcumin on the ER is not very clear at the moment. In our opinion, it represents a major challenge for the future. Indeed, a growing number of studies show the key role of this organelle in the development of numerous PN (diabetes, alcohol, chemotherapy, genetic mutations...). Thus, because of its numerous biological properties, curcumin reduces tissue damage or improves tissue repair (nerve, muscle, DRG) in many PN. These effects are also reflected at the behavioral level by reducing the signs of pain, improving sensory and motor recovery. However, despite a large number of pre-clinical studies (both in vitro and in vivo) on the subject and a large amount of laboratory evidence of curcumin's efficacy, studies in humans are sorely lacking. Indeed, to date, only four clinical studies have been specifically conducted in humans in the field of PN. These studies, although encouraging, are sometimes carried out on too few subjects and therefore make it difficult to objectify the use of curcumin clinically for PN. However, the large number of studies on inflammatory pain represents hope for the future use of this molecule for the treatment of neuropathies. We therefore believe that the advent of new curcumin formulations represents a key milestone in the treatment of PN in humans.

Sirtuins functions in central nervous system cells under neurological disorders

Jing Yan, 1 Xiaole Tang, 2 Zhi-qiang Zhou, 1 Jie Zhang, 1 Yilin Zhao, 1 Shiyong Li,[1],* and Ailin Luo[1],*
Author information Article notes Copyright and License information PMC Disclaimer

Abstract

The sirtuins (SIRTs), a class of NAD+ -dependent deacylases, contain seven SIRT family members in mammals, from SIRT1 to SIRT7. Extensive studies have revealed that SIRT proteins regulate virous cell functions. Central nervous system (CNS) decline resulted in progressive cognitive impairment, social and physical abilities dysfunction. Therefore, it is of vital importance to have a better understanding of potential target to promote homeostasis of CNS. SIRTs have merged as the underlying regulating factors of the process of neurological disorders. In this review, we profile multiple functions of SIRT proteins in different cells during brain function and under CNS injury.

Keywords: sirtuins, central nervous syste, neuron, microglia, astrocyte, oligodendrocyte

Introduction

SIRTs in mammals are a class of proteins that possess NAD + dependent deacetylase activity or ADP-ribosyltransferase activity varies from SIRT1 to SIRT7. These SIRTs are present in different tissue and subcellular localization: SIRT1 and SIRT2 are expressed in the nucleus and cytoplasm, whereas SIRT3, SIRT4, and SIRT5 are mitochondrial, and SIRT6 and SIRT7 localized only in the nucleus (Cai et al., 2016). The initial studies found Sir2 protein contributes to lifespan extension in yeasts, worms and flies in which Sir2 and its orthologs mediated caloric restriction-induced extension of lifespan in certain genetic backgrounds (Li et al., 2007). However, mice overexpressing SIRT1 did not show lifespan extension. Striking, whole-body SIRT6 transgenic mice showed lifespan extension in males (Zorrilla-Zubilete et al., 2018). Later studies indicated SIRTs 'protect brain function in virous mammalian models. Recent evidence showed that SIRTs exert anti-aging and neuroprotective effect through regulating diverse cell functions and responses to stressors (Herskovits and Guarente, 2014). Herein we review multiple functions of SIRT proteins during maintaining normal cellular function in central nervous system.

SIRT1 in neurons in central nervous system

Sirtuin 1 (SIRT1) is a member of the nicotinamide adenine dinucleotide (NAD)+-dependent class III histone deacetylases, which is the studied one among the SIRT family (Gomes et al., 2018). Mounting Data suggest SIRT1 to be an important factor involved in a vast physiological and pathological role in brain through modulating variety of molecular signaling pathways essential for central nerves system homeostasis and normal brain function. In mammalian cells, SIRT1 located in nucleus and cytoplasm. Within the nucleus, SIRT1 regulates transcription process through promoting histone deacetylation and modulating DNA methylation. Within the cytoplasm, SIRT1 participates in regulating various cellular processes, such as cell apoptosis, oxidative stress, autophagy, endoplasmic reticulum stress and mitophagy.

Some studies suggest that cytoplasm-localized SIRT1 promotes apoptosis, while the anti-apoptotic effect attributes to the nuclear-localized SIRT1. Research indicated that SIRT1 plays a pivotal role in alleviating apoptosis. Upregulated SIRT1 alleviated manganese-induced neuronal apoptosis through activation of FOXO3a, and activated expression of SIRT1 also alleviating the apoptosis of mouse hippocampal neurons (HT22) cells through facilitating the deacetylation and phosphorylation of FOXO3a (Zhao et al., 2021a). Mostly, SIRT1 exerts neuroprotective effect through reducing apoptosis. However, nicotinamide, a pharmacological inhibitor of SIRT1, enhances neuronal survival and reduces apoptosis during acute anoxic injury, implying the benefit of SIRT1 deficiency, seemly indicate that SIRT1 might play a detrimental role (Chong and Maiese, 2008). Pharmacological or genetically downregulated SIRT1 significantly reduced ERK1/2 activation and promoted apoptotic neuron death both *in vitro* and *in vivo* of traumatic brain injury models (Zhao et al., 2012). SIRT1 deficiency in neuron leads to the acetylation of p53, a critical transcriptional factor that controls apoptotic programs and also the first nonhistone deacetylation target for SIRT1, thereby instigating neuronal death in cerebral ischemic stroke mice (Chen et al., 2014).

SIRT 1 has a vital role in autophagy stimulation through deacetylating autophagy-related proteins including FoxO, Atg5, Atg7, and Atg8 (Hariharan et al., 2010). Also, SIRT1 is a major deacetylase for BECN1 K430 and K437, which form multiple protein complexes participating in autophagy (Xu and Wan, 2022). Oxidative stress could decrease SIRT1 enzymatic activity and protein stability through promoting SIRT1 cysteinyl carbonylation on Cys482, and SIRT1-deficient cells are more sensitive to exogenous H_2O_2 that could induce autophagy (Zhou et al., 2022a). SIRT1 activation plays a pivotal role protecting against prion-induced neuronal death through regulating autophagy process (Jeong et al., 2013). In a cardiac arrest-related brain injury, researchers used a SIRT1 loss of function approach and found that suppression of SIRT1 compromised the neuroprotection by mild hypothermia treatment both *in vivo* and *in vitro* through mediating autophagic flux, they came up with the idea that FOXO1, a transcription factor binds to several consensus sites on the SIRT1 promoter and enables its transcription, might be the upstream of SIRT1 in this model, and further investigation is warranted (Wei et al., 2019).

Accumulating evidence has indicated that SIRT1 function is tightly related to axon genesis and neurite outgrowth. SIRT1 deficiency could cause synaptic plasticity impairment and cognitive dysfunction (Cai et al., 2016). SIRT1 regulates transcription factors, including nuclear factor-E2-related factor 2 (Nrf2), a major regulator in antioxidant defenses, to exert a neuroprotective effect by inducing neurite outgrowth in Neuro-2a cells (Duangjan et al., 2021), peroxisome proliferator-activated receptor coactivator-1α (PGC-1α), a fasting-induced transcriptional coactivator recruited during PPAR stimulation, to restore neuronal network disconnection through reversing synaptic failure in hippocampal neuron *in vitro* (Panes et al., 2020). In neonatal propofol exposure experiment, SIRT1 was tightly related to synaptic plasticity and neuronal excitability in the hippocampal CA1 region (Ma et al., 2022).

SIRT1 also take parts in physiological and pathological process correlated to neuronal cell damage such as oxidative stress, metabolic disorders and calcium homeostasis. It has been reported that SIRT1 counteracts the activation of acetyl-STAT3 (Lys685) and increase neural senescence and affects locomotor behavior (Liu et al., 2021a). SIRT1/PGC-1α pathway relieving neuronal oxidative stress through activating mitochondrial biogenesis against Aβ1-42 oligomer-induced oxidative stress (Yin et al., 2021a). As SIRT1 mediated caloric restriction, study on unhealthy-diet-induced learning and memory loss found that biogenesis related genes SIRT1 and PGC1α upregulated along with reversed high-glucose-induced oxidized cellular status, mitochondrial membrane impairment, insulin signaling inhibition and neuron damage in high-fat and high-fructose feed mice (Liu et al., 2017). Compelling investment revealed that SIRT1 provides neuroprotection by promoting calcium regulation in neurons (Stoyas et al., 2020). In a PD mice model, SIRT1 was found downregulated in neuron, which leading to FOXO1 acetylation upregulation, and subsequently increased the transcription level of type A monoamine oxidase (MAO-A), an enzyme primarily engaged in catalyzing the oxidative deamination of NA and 5-HT and leading to inactivation and degradation of both monoamines. Activation SIRT1 by resveratrol restored brain NA and 5-HT levels and attenuates the depressive-like behavior (Li et al., 2020a). The effect of SIRT1 changing the acetylation status of BMAL1 and PER2 and further affecting their activity and stability respectively, is involved in the metabolism mechanism of circadian machinery (Asher et al., 2008). Later, Aras et al. provide *in vivo* evidence that SIRT1 deficiency in neurons within the hypothalamic ventromedial nucleus are more prone to develop metabolic imbalance (Ramadori et al., 2011). What's more, they also found that SIRT1 in neurons within the hypothalamic ventromedial nucleus convey photic inputs to entrain the biochemical and metabolic action of insulin in skeletal muscle in mice (Aras et al., 2019).

In hypoxia-ischemia rat, SIRT1 expression significantly reduced in neuron, and was related to the increased ER stress and neurotoxicity due to its action in the modulation of a wide variety of signaling pathways involved in neuroprotection (Carloni et al., 2014). In our previous studies, SIRT1 overexpression could reduce tau acetylation and thus preserve cognitive function in mice following anesthesia and surgery (Yan et al., 2020). Later, our team investigate the role of neuronal SIRT1 in developing mice exposed to volatile anesthetic sevoflurane, we found that SIRT1 epigeneticlly regulated the activity of MeCP2 and CREB, therefor affect the expression of BDNF, which is a vital factor for normal neuronal function (Tang et al., 2020).

SIRT1 in microglia in central nervous system

Microglia are immune cells of the resident macrophages in the brain, which is continually involved in surveillance of the brain parenchyma, and providing as the first line of defense against disease-causing pathogenic stimuli. Mountings of findings indicated that SIRT1 deficiency could injury normal function of microglia (Meng et al., 2020). Mitochondria dysfunction linked neurodegeneration and neuroinflammation *via* coordinating innate and adaptive immune responses, and initiate and promoted the activation of microglia through increase reactive oxygen species (ROS). It has been reported that SIRT1 regulates PGC-1α by increasing its expression and decreasing its acetylation in microglia at least in part rescued mitochondria injury, decreased ROS production, and reduced neuroinflammatory response which ultimately ameliorated the cognitive dysfunction in chronic cerebral hypoperfusion models *in vivo* and *in vitro* (Zhao et al., 2021b). PGC-1α, a major regulator of ROS metabolism and mitochondria biogenesis, has also been proved to be downstream of SIRT1 in post-neonatal hypoxic–ischemic encephalopathy rat (Xie et al., 2021). HMGB1/NF-kB pathway also might be downstream of SIRT1 to inhibit microglia activation and proinflammatory cytokines release in subarachnoid hemorrhage rats and LPS treated BV2 cells (Wang et al., 2019; Zhang et al., 2020a; Li et al., 2020b).

Chronic and persistent activation of microglia has been proved to drive cells in the central nerves system to senescence phenotype through senescence-associated beta-galactosidase (SA β-gal) activity upregulation, growth arrest, and senescence-associated secretory phenotypes (SASPs) which involves uncontrolled secretion of proinflammatory cytokines, which exhibit detrimental effects on cells (Hardeland, 2019). SIRT1 was reduced in aging brain and associated with the impairment of learning and memory (Chaudhuri et al., 2013; Meng et al., 2020). In our previous work, we found that SIRT1 expression significantly decreased in anesthesia and surgery treated aged mice, and upregulated SIRT1 could significantly reduce microglia activation-related neuroinflammation and ameliorated cognitive impairment through regulating the expression of DNMT1 and ac-NF-κB (Yan et al., 2019). Our result is consistent with a previous study that SIRT1 deficiency in microglia contribute to aging and neurodegeneration-related cognition decline, importantly, in this article, they proved that SIRT1 exert neuroprotection through hypomethylating the specific CpG sites on IL-1β proximal promoter which is a classic inflammatory factor (Cho et al., 2015). Later, our team investigated SIRT1/NF-κB signaling in developing mice, as expected, we found that SIRT1 overexpression inhibited microglial activation and improved the long-term cognitive function through decreasing the expression of ac-NF-κB (Tang et al., 2021). In early 2005, Li Gan and his group have indicated that overexpression of SIRT1 deacetylase increased acetylation of RelA/p65 at lysine 310 and regulates the NF-κB pathway in amyloid-β peptides treated primary microglia (Meng et al., 2020). Recent research confirmed that in BV2 cells, reduced SIRT1 expression caused an increased inflammatory response in microglia termed as M1 polarization and promoted microglial migration (Yin et al., 2021b), and suppressed acetylation of NF-κB p65 subunit by SIRT1 in BV-2 microglia decreased the inflammatory factors, including TNF-α and IL-6 (Qin et al., 2020; Zhu et al., 2020). Besides, SIRT1 exerted protection against hypoxic-derived neuronal damage through regulating NF-κB (Merlo et al., 2020). And activated SIRT1/FOXO1 pathway could also reduce microglia activation and inflammatory response (Zhang et al., 2021a). SIRT1 down-regulated the level of Ac-NFκB expression and then suppressed the expression of pro-inflammatory cytokines, accompanied by the decreased activation of microglia, to withhold the cognitive function in mice (Pan et al., 2018). Furthermore, downregulated SIRT1 level prevented M2 microglial polarization and promote motor and nonmotor deficits in Parkinson's disease (PD) mice (Yang et al., 2021).

The anti-inflammatory effect of SIRT1 has also been explored in several neurodegenerative diseases. In Parkinson's disease models, SIRT1 signaling pathway is involved in NLRP3 inflammasome activation in microglia (Zheng et al., 2021), that has been proved again in an subarachnoid hemorrhage mice model in which SIRT1 not only involved in microglia activation, but also M2 microglial polarization (Zhang et al., 2021b). In aluminum chloride treated mice, SIRT1 regulated DDX3X-NLRP3 Inflammasome signaling pathway (Hao et al., 2021). Other substrate of SIRT1 such as NF-κB has been found changed and involved in microglial polarization in Parkinson's disease models (Yang et al., 2021). In Alzheimer's disease models, SIRT1 directly interacted with and deacetylated TFEB at lysine residue 116 to enhanced lysosomal function and fAβ degradation, thus attenuating amyloid plaque deposition in APP/PS1 transgenic mice (Bao et al., 2016).

SIRT1 has been found neuroprotective in other neurological disorders such as microgliopathic pain, which might be stimulated by activated microglia induced abnormal discharge of neurons, *via* its anti-inflammatory effect (Wen et al., 2021); and radiation-induced brain injury, in which SIRT1 exert protective effect through reducing oxidative stress damage, inflammation and microglial infiltration (Liu et al., 2021b); and chronic unpredictable mild stress mice model, in which SIRT1 signaling exerted antidepressant effect through modulating NLRP3 inflammasome deactivation (Tong et al., 2020); and brain injury in epilepsy and acute ethanol intoxication, in which SIRT1 prevented astrocytes and microglia activation, as well as inhibition of oxidative stress (Khan et al., 2018; Kong et al., 2020); and LPS treated neonatal mice, in which SIRT1/Nrf2 signaling pathway activation reduced LPS-induced oxidative stress damage, acute neuroinflammation, and apoptotic neurodegeneration (Shah et al., 2017). Researches also demonstrated that SIRT1 deficiency in microglia caused neuroinflammation, subsequently impaired neuronal function through apoptosis, autophagy, et al. (Liu et al., 2019).

SIRT1 in astrocytes in central nervous system

Astrocytes perform various functions in central nerves system including immunity modulation, transmitter uptake and regulation, brain structures support, blood-brain barrier permeability regulation. Downregulation of SIRT1 is reported to be related with astrocytes activation in PD model, AD model and traumatic brain injury model (Scuderi et al., 2014; Abd El-Fatah et al., 2021; Zhang et al., 2021c; Har-Even et al., 2021; Yang et al., 2022). HIV-associated neurocognitive disorders presented in almost 50% of the infected individuals, it was founded downregulated SIRT1 expression in the HIV Tg rats with a concomitant increase in astrocyte marker (Hu et al., 2017). Astrocytic SIRT1 inhibition significantly increased the acetylation of forehead box protein O4, decreased the expression of superoxide dismutase two and catalase, and increased reactive oxygen species production *in vitro* (Cheng et al., 2014). Confocal imaging showed that SIRT1 upregulated by resveratrol increased the expression of LC3 in astrocytes around the lesion site after injury in traumatic brain injury mice (Zhang et al., 2019a). In brain injury model, elevated SIRT1 levels by resveratrol significantly increases the level of p-ERK but reduces the levels of p-JNK and p-p38 protein, thus attenuated astrocyte activation (Li et al., 2017). Also, SIRT1 upregulation was accompanied with downregulated mRNA expression of pro-inflammatory cytokines, including TNF-α and IL-1β, decreased activation of astrocytes and ameliorated blood-brain barrier disruption in ischemic brain of mice (Li et al., 2020c).

As astrocyte activation precedes extracellular Aβ deposition, an AD research focused on astrocyte function, and they found that SIRT1 could enhance the ability of astrocytes to clear Aβ, and subsequently essentially delay the formation of amyloid deposits *via* deacetylating several lysosome-related proteins and upregulate lysosome number (Li et al., 2018). In chronic cerebral hypoperfusion rat model, AMPK/SIRT1 signaling was reduced along with increased expression of STAT3/NF-κB pathway (Li et al., 2020d). Other substrate of SIRT1 in astrocytes has been revealed. SIRT1 plays a protective role against astrocyte activation through interaction with Dnajb1 and modulate the deacetylation and ubiquitination of Dnajb1 *in vivo* and *in vitro* model of traumatic brain injury (Zhang et al., 2022). In cerebral ischemia/reperfusion injury model, SIRT1 directly mediated the PGC-1α/PPARγ pathway in astrocytes, attenuated oxidative stress injury and therefore reversed the neurological deficit (Zhou et al., 2022b).

SIRT1 in oligodendrocytes in central nervous system

Oligodendrocyte precursors differentiate into mature myelin forming oligodendrocytes to preserve the balance between demyelination and remyelination, which keep the myelin sheath renewal and the axons in a normal status, thus support neuron nutrition in the central nervous system (Prozorovski et al., 2019; Hisahara et al., 2021). As mature and terminally differentiated cells that form myelin sheaths around axons, oligodendrocyte are found predominantly, but not exclusively, in CNS white matter, and could produce myelin sheaths that allow "saltatory" action potential propagation, therefor greatly increases conduction velocity, speeding the efficiency of communication between CNS neurons (Zhou et al., 2021). In an exercise training and dietary fat interplay mice model, SIRT1, PGC-1α and antioxidant enzymes were increased and contribute to mitochondrial activity in oligodendroglia in response to higher levels of reactive oxygen species (Yoon et al., 2016). SIRT1 regulated oligodendrocyte regeneration *via* deacetylating retinoblastoma in the Rb/E2F1 complex, leading to E2F1 dissociation in neonatal brain injury mice (Jablonska et al., 2016). In a mouse model of multiple sclerosis, increased oligodendrocyte generation and decreased apoptosis were consistent with increased SIRT1 expression (Mojaverrostami et al., 2020). It was observed that SIRT1 co-localizes with surviving oligodendrocytes in multiple sclerosis plaques, then the research group found a significant reduction in phospho-SIRT1 and SIRT1 expression during oligodendrocytes differentiation, associated with decreased expression of H3K9me3 and increased cyclin D1 (Tatomir et al., 2020). Taken together, SIRT1 promoted oligodendrocytes differentiation and regeneration in the CNS.

SIRT2 in central nervous system cells

SIRT2 is predominantly cytosolic and shuttle between the cytoplasm and nucleus. Several studies indicated an important role of SIRT2 in cognitive and brain function. SIRT2 localized to the outer and juxtanodal loops in the myelin sheath and has a counterbalancing role on oligodendroglial differentiation (Li et al., 2007). Fang N found that SIRT2 translocated into the nuclei, epigeneticly downregulated PDGFRα expression and facilitate the differentiation of oligodendroglial cell line (Fang et al., 2019).

ATP homeostasis in axons is highly vulnerable to bioenergetic failure, and is required in neuron function. *In vivo* research revealed that of SIRT2 transcellular oligodendrocyte-to-axon delivery enhances ATP production by deacetylating mitochondrial proteins and enhanced axonal energy in mice (Chamberlain et al., 2021). SIRT2 is highly expressed in oligodendrocytes and be released within exosomes. Still, there are few researches found SIRT2 expressed in neurons. Genetic or pharmacologic SIRT2 inhibition reduced sterol levels *via* decreased nuclear SREBP-2 trafficking and showed neuroprotective effect in a striatal neuron model of HD (Luthi-Carter et al., 2010).

On the other hand, SIRT2 inhibition has been proved beneficial in some neurodegenerative mouse model. Pais TF reported, for the first time, that SIRT2 is also expressed in microglia and the absence of SIRT2 enhanced microglia activation associated with a proinflammatory phenotype induced by LPS in BV2 cells (Pais et al., 2013). Compelling evidence indicated that SIRT2 accumulates in several microglia models. SIRT2 increased lipopolysaccharide-induced microglial activation *in vivo* and *in vitro* through regulation of MAKP signaling and inflammatory response including a major inflammation transcription regulator, the p65 subunit of NF-kB (Chen et al., 2015a; Jiao et al., 2020),besides, SIRT2 showed potential effect on intracellular ATP levels through poly (ADP-ribose) polymerase (PARP) activation in microglia cell line (Li et al., 2013). Animal study showed that SIRT2 also promote sevoflurane-induced learning and memory deficits in the developing rat brain. SIRT2 inhibitor, AK7, pretreatment protected against sevoflurane-mediated cognitive impairments possibly by enhancing the proportion of M2-phenotype microglia (Wu et al., 2020). However, AK7, the brain-permeable SIRT2 inhibitor, which showed neuroprotective effect in neurodegenerative disease including Parkinson's disease and Huntington's disease by protecting dopaminergic neurons against aSyn-induced neurotoxicity *in vitro* and promotes long-term survival of dopaminergic neurons *in vivo*, does not show beneficial effects in amyotrophic lateral sclerosis and cerebral ischemia mouse model (Chen et al., 2015b). Furthermore, studies have reported that AK7 is not beneficial under conditions where the control of the microglial response is crucial for neuronal survival, and the anti-inflammatory properties of SIRT2 through post-translational deacetylation of p65 might be a underlying mechanism (Romeo-Guitart et al., 2018). Not only in microglia, in rat primary astrocytes, SIRT2 inhibition partly induced cellular senescence through increase senescence-associated β-galactosidase (SA-β-gal) activity, senescence-associated secretory phenotypes and cell cycle-related proteins (Bang et al., 2019).

SIRT3 in neurons in central nervous system

Sirtuin-3 (SIRT3), localized in the mitochondria, is a NAD +-dependent deacetylase. SIRT3 exerts protection against the progression of cognitive dysfunction through regulates mitochondrial energy metabolism, antioxidant mechanisms, inflammation, autophagy, and cell death processes *via* targeting of the involved enzymes (Almalki et al., 2021). Mitochondria are small double-membrane organelles which could provide energy for cellular functions. Mitochondrial dysfunction has reported as a significant determinant in brain dysfunction pathophysiological processes (Song et al., 2013). SIRT3 can deacetylate and activate LKB1 (liver kinase B1), and active LKB1 can phosphorylate AMPK to activate AMPK (Liu et al., 2020). In ischemic-injured PC12 cells, promoting SIRT3/AMPK pathway significantly increased cell survival, decreased apoptosis rate and increased the mitochondrial autophagy (Li et al., 2021). It has been reported that increased SIRT3 providing neuroprotective effects *via* enhancing mitochondrial function, increase neuron survival and decrease the number of apoptotic neurons in cerebral ischemia rat through activation of the SIRT3/AMPK/ mTOR pathway (Liu et al., 2020). In addition, SIRT3 alleviated cell death and promoted cell viability of the HT22 cells through preservation of mitochondrial function (Lin et al., 2021). Cerebral ischemia-reperfusion injury caused neuron apoptosis, SIRT3 overexpression attenuated neuron apoptosis possibly through blocking caspase-9-dependent mitochondrial apoptotic signals and suppressed mitochondrial fission *via* activating the Wnt/β-catenin pathway *in vitro* and *in vivo* (Zhao et al., 2018).

SIRT3 played a positive role in promoting autophagy in HT22 cells to resist from the neurotoxicity induced by Aβ1–42 oligomers through increasing Beclin-1 and LC3-II expression, as well as led to the p62 expression (Zhang et al., 2020b). In a subarachnoid hemorrhage mice model, SIRT3 exerted anti-apoptotic effect on neuron through deacetylated SOD to decrease neuron lose (Zhang et al., 2019b). In Aβ42 treated APPTG mice, SIRT3 activity and expression was found to be decreased and be associated with hippocampal neuron cell apoptosis and cognition deficit (Liu et al., 2021c). Besides, SIRT3 has been reported as neuroprotective in ALS models (Harlan et al., 2020). However, the underline mechanism of SIRT3 in these processes still needs further investment. In a high-fat diet mice model, the hippocampus plasticity was reduced and spatial learning function was compromised, SIRT3 upregulation could decrease hippocampal neuron oxidative stress and apoptosis to attenuates high-fat diet-associated cognitive dysfunction through acetylate antioxidative MnSOD (Shi et al., 2018). In an ischemia research, SIRT3 SUMOylation triggered by SENP1 subsequently results in increased levels of COX1, SOD2, and IDH2 protein acetylation, which caused oxidative stress and mitochondrial dysfunction *in vitro* and *in vivo* (Cai et al., 2021).

In a study of SIRT3-depleted mice, the behavioral phenotypes have been explored, they found that locomotion, anxiety, and recent memory of the mice remain normal, but the remote memory was impaired, this consist with impaired long-term potentiation in the anterior cingulate cortex which might due to neuronal loss (Kim et al., 2019). It has been reported that SIRT3 reduction caused aggravated GABAergic neuron loss and neuronal network hyperexcitability in Sirt3+/-AppPs1 mice (Cheng et al., 2020). Besides, SIRT3 was found increased in substantia nigra after physical exercise which might be related to an increase in expression of the protective Ang 1-7/Mas axis and inhibition of the Ang II/AT1 axis (Munoz et al., 2018). Although these results suggest that SIRT3 is protective in neuronal function in various manners including neuronal apoptosis, autophagy, mitochondrial function preservation, neuronal network hyperexcitability, future investigations are necessary to confirm the underline signaling pathways.

Research on cardiomyopathy revealed that PGC-1α plays a role in moderating SIRT3, which in turn deacetylates enzymes to control antioxidants and the metabolization of mitochondrial energy

(Zhu et al., 2020). Similarly, PGC-1α/SIRT3 pathway have been reported neuroprotective in hippocampus by preventing damage to mitochondria and preventing cell apoptosis and neuron loss (Cheng et al., 2021). As we have discussed in 1.1, SIRT1 has been proved to be downstream of SIRT1, thus SIRT1/PGC-1alpha/SIRT3 pathway might play an essential role in mitochondrial dysfunction, oxidative stress and related neurological deficits. (Cheng et al., 2021).

SIRT3 in microlgia in central nervous system

SIRT3 overexpression in mouse primary microglia prevented the microglia senescence through decreasing the expression of mitochondrial antioxidant enzymes (Thangaraj et al., 2021). In a study of PD cell model, they found that decreased expression of SIRT3 underlines the pathological process of microglia activation resulted oxidative stress injury, membrane potential depolarization and mPTP opening mediated cell apoptosis in dopaminergic neurons (Jiang et al., 2019). In addition, SIRT3 exerted an anti-apoptotic effect in LPS-treated BV2 cells through suppressing the transcription of SRV2 *via* the Mst1-JNK pathway and thus suppressed mitochondrial fission. (Zhou and Jiang, 2019) Besides, Yun Yuan and his group found that SIRT3 expression could be inhibited by Notch signaling pathway interference in microglia, and that SIRT1 and Notch synergistically regulate microglia activation including TNF-α production (Guo et al., 2021). Several SIRT3 substrates have been reported involved in mitochondrial biogenesis and dynamism pathways dependent pathological mechanisms (Liu et al., 2021d). In mouse primary microglial, overexpression of SIRT3 prevented HIV Trans-activator of transcription mediated imbalance of mitochondrial oxidative stress and induction of senescence phenotype (Thangaraj et al., 2021).

In an ischemia animal model, SIRT3 expression was found to be increased in macrophages, and increased SIRT3 promoted microglial N9 cells migration by upregulating CX3CR1 (Cao et al., 2019). Activated microglia caused uncontrolled production of ROS which forms an important basis for microglia-mediated neurodegeneration and associated cognition deficit. It was reported that microglial SIRT3 upregulation facilitates the increase in Foxo3a expression and its nuclear localization to carry out its antioxidant-mediated attenuation of ROS. The researchers reassured SIRT3 as the upstream regulator of Foxo3a in microglia using Sirt3-/- mouse (Rangarajan et al., 2015). In 2021, Yu-Qing Wu and his group found that SIRT3 suppressed hippocampal neuroinflammation and exert protection in anesthesia/surgery-induced cognitive decline in aged mice through ameliorating the anesthesia/surgery-induced mitochondrial oxidative stress response, microglia activation and neuroinflammation (Liu et al., 2021d). In a study of Alzheimer's Disease, researchers found that SIRT3 deficiency caused microglia activation following exposure to a combination of high glucose and palmitic acid using SIRT3 shRNA Lentiviral particles in BV2 cells, and enhanced microglial and endothelial interactions which may leading to BBB breakdown, and thus caused cognitive dysfunction, however, the mechanism of SIRT3 deficiency under microglial and endothelial interactions has not been further exacerbated (Tyagi et al., 2021).

SIRT3 in astrocytes and oligodendrocytes in central nervous system

It was reported that SIRT3 mediated the inhibitory effect of adjudin in astrocyte activation and glial scar formation in mouse model of transient middle cerebral artery occlusion and in primary astrocytes (Yang et al., 2017). Knockdown of SIRT3 using specific siRNA (Si-Sirt3) partially reserved the effects of AMPAR antagonist on neuronal injury and BBB function *in vitro* neurovascular unit (NVU) system including neurons, astrocytes, and brain microvascular endothelial cells (Chen et al., 2021). what's more, SIRT3 also act as a factor regulating non-cell-autonomous neuronal death through glia. SIRT3 overexpression suppressed oxidative stress-induced neuronal toxicity in SH-SY5Y cells while SIRT3 deficiency promoted rotenone- or H_2O_2-induced neuronal toxicity in differentiated SH-SY5Y cells (**Lee et al., 2021**).

Seldom studies focusing on investigating the role of SIRT3 in astrocytes and oligodendrocytes. Further study is required to determine roles of SIRT3 in the two types of glia cells.

SIRT4/5 in central nervous system cells

SIRT4 and SIRT5 both localize in mitochondria. SIRT4 is an ADP-ribosyltransferase whereas SIRT5 is a desuccinylase and demalonylase with weak deacetylase activity (**Kida and Goligorsky, 2016**). In hepatic encephalopathy, overexpression SIRT4 in astrocyte inhibited GDH2 activity and restored mitochondrial respiration (**Drews et al., 2020**), which suggests SIRT4 exert a protective effect in astrocyte. In an AD model, the expression of SIRT5 was significantly decreased, along with suppressed autophagy in neuron. Overexpression of SIRT5 in glia cells repressed microglia and astrocyte activation, and restored oxidative stress-induced brain damage (**Wu et al., 2021**). Currently investigations focused on SIRT4 and SIRT5 in CNS are rare.

Go to:

SIRT6 in central nervous system cells

SIRT6 is a chromatin-associated protein that stabilizes genomes and prevents cell premature senescence. In mice cortical and hippocampal primary neurons, SIRT6 is closely related with synaptic function, neuronal maturation and neuronal survival (**Cardinale et al., 2015**). Another study indicated that SIRT6 levels affect synaptic plasticity and neuronal survival *via* regulating Akt-GSK3β signaling, moreover, upregulated SIRT6 is related to depression-like behavior, which indicated that SIRT6 might exert neurotoxic effect on neuron (**Mao et al., 2017**) Another study on PD suggest that SIRT6 plays a pathogenic and pro-inflammatory role (Nicholatos et al., 2018). On the other hand, decreased SIRT6 expression has been found in the spinal cord of amyotrophic lateral sclerosis (ALS) patients, enhancing the activity or expression of SIRT6 abrogates its neurotoxicity in cell culture models of ALS (Harlan et al., 2020). In an ischemic stroke model, LPS-stimulated inflammatory response in primary mouse microglia can be inhibited by SIRT6 activation (He et al., 2021). The dual effect of SIRT6 in central nervous system may due to different pathological context. Currently it is not fully elucidated whether SIRT6 is protective in CNS.

SIRT7 in central nervous system cells

SIRT7 is the only SIRT protein localized predominantly in the nucleoli (Wang et al., 2020). In cerebral ischemia/reperfusion injury cell model, overexpression of SIRT7 protect neurons possibly through regulating p53-mediated proapoptotic signaling pathway (Lv et al., 2017). SIRT7 knockdown mice proved slight protective effect through regulating cell differentiation and cytokine production *via* reducing peripheral IFN-γ production and failed accumulation of regulatory T cells in the CNS. Besides, SIRT7 promoted adult-born neurons survival but had no effect on hippocampal neurons proliferation (Burg et al., 2018). Future investigations are need to clarify the SIRT7 function in CNS.

www.ingramcontent.com/pod-product-compliance
Lightning Source LLC
Chambersburg PA
CBHW071010250726

48653CB00005B/1571